MAKING THE CHEMOTHERAPY DECISION

D1215760

MAKING THE CHEMOTHERAPY DECISION

DAVID DRUM

Foreword by
Michael B. Van Scoy-Mosher, M.D., M.A.

Lowell House
Los Angeles

Contemporary Books
Chicago

Library of Congress Cataloging-in-Publication Data

Drum, David E.
    Making the chemotherapy decision / David Drum.
        p.   cm.
    Includes bibliographical references and index.
    ISBN 1-56565-445-5
    1. Cancer—Chemotherapy.   2. Cancer—Popular works.
    I. Title.
  RC271.C5D79 1996
  616.99' 4061—dc20   96-3659
                                                  CIP

Requests for such permissions should be addressed to:
Lowell House
2029 Century Park East, Suite 3290
Los Angeles, CA 90067

Lowell House books can be purchased at special discounts when ordered in bulk for premiums and special sales. Contact Department JH at the address above.

Publisher: Jack Artenstein
General Manager, Lowell House Adult: Bud Sperry
Managing Editor: Maria Magallanes
Text design: Kate Mueller / Electric Dragon Productions

Manufactured in the United States of America
10 9 8 7 6 5 4 3 2

The more serious the illness, the more important it is for you to fight back, mobilizing all your resources — spiritual, emotional, intellectual, physical.

NORMAN COUSINS

To my children,
Leanne, Amy, and Justin Drum

Acknowledgments

First and foremost, the author would like to acknowledge the significant contribution made by the insightful men and women who completed chemotherapy treatment, and who agreed to share their experiences and successes with the readers of this book. In addition, thanks are due to several individuals within the medical community who generously shared their information and expertise: Kim Margolin, M.D., City of Hope National Medical Center, Duarte, California; Paul Coluzzi, M.D., M.P.H., Regional Medical Director, Vitas Healthcare Corporation of California, Anaheim Hills, California; Diane R. Morrison, L.C.S.W., Director of TQM Services, USC/Norris Comprehensive Cancer Center and Hospital, Los Angeles; Sharon Steingass, Clinical Director, USC/Norris Comprehensive Cancer Center and Hospital; Phil Manly, chaplain, USC/Norris Comprehensive Cancer Center and Hospital; Janine McDonough, director, Positive Image Center, City of Hope National Medical Center; Skip Shoden, CCN, New Health, Santa Monica, California; Denise Jamin, Ph.D., assistant professor of pharmacy, University of Southern California, Los Angeles; personal finance writer Laura Meyers; Cecilia Olkowski, M.B.A., director of cancer control, American Cancer Society, Oakland, California; and the many other individuals within the National Institute of Health's Cancer Information Service and the American Cancer Society who responded to my many requests for information. I would also like to acknowledge the special contribution of Dr. Michael Van Scoy-Mosher, who critically reviewed this book and provided timely and useful advice.

CONTENTS

Introduction

MORE THAN 300,000 AMERICANS ARE CURED OF CANCER EVERY year. Of the major chronic illnesses, such as heart disease, diabetes, emphysema, and cerebrovacular disease, cancer is the only one that can truly be cured. Yet, because of the remarkable degree of misinformation and fear existing in the minds of many, the diagnosis of cancer is still often felt to be tantamount to a death sentence. Believing a diagnosis equals fatality or a terminal condition can itself so weaken the spirit that indeed it becomes a self-fulfilling prophecy. It is the panic that cancer brings to mind that immobilizes many from being vigorous about applying preventative and early detection methods to themselves; if properly applied, these could reduce the annual mortality from cancer by about 200,000 people.

Making the Chemotherapy Decision has been written for those who choose to fight, for those who choose to use all the forces available to overcome their cancer. These include their own internal capabilities of reasoning and psychic energy, as well as all the external contributions of modern medical science.

Making the Chemotherapy Decision is for those who, when faced with the diagnosis of cancer, see it as a challenge against which they are willing to apply their maximal efforts toward victory. They understand that the optimal treatment of cancer can be likened to the solving of a jigsaw puzzle: Many different and complex pieces must be precisely integrated. The best chance for cure comes from understanding that each "piece" is essential, whether that piece be surgery, chemotherapy, or a healthy mental attitude toward therapy.

The first step in this journey is your reeducation about cancer. "Cancer" should not be viewed as a single disease, but as a collection of more than one hundred quite distinct illnesses, each with its own causes, treatments, and likely outcomes. In a given individual, the type of cancer is further identified as being in a certain "stage" based on its size, location, and degree of involvement of associated lymph nodes and other anatomic structures. Only from a thorough evaluation of the type and stage of a particular cancer can one even begin to develop a sense of the indicated and proper treatment, as well as the possible prognosis, for an individual patient. Furthermore, even with the same type and stage of cancer, different patients can have radically different results of therapy and overall outcome.

Thus, even with a known type of cancer and a specific stage, all that can intelligently be given as a prognosis for an individual is a likely *range of possibilities,* and not a precise prediction for that person. It is not possible to apply statistical probabilities from a group of patients to any one patient. If some in a particular situation die from their disease within a short time, while others in the identical situation live for many years, and some are cured, what has made the difference between them? Was it the medical treatment? Was it luck? Was it some combination of these and other, unknown factors? Whatever it might be, you owe it to yourself to do whatever can be done to give yourself the best chance for recovery.

Obviously, then, it is an absurdity to generalize about what it might mean to "have cancer," or even to have "lung cancer." Though it can be stressful to become intimately involved in the details, it is vital to learn and understand the specifics of your own situation, enabling you to comprehend the reasoning behind the treatment plan and to become a true partner with your physician in the development and application of the plan. Not every patient is really comfortable with and desirous of learning the details of his or her own diagnosis. Such patients then should endeavor to develop a relationship with a physician who they can trust and in whom they have great confidence that he or she will offer a plan that is in their best interest.

The treatments of cancer can themselves be an ordeal. But they can become far more tolerable under the right conditions. First of all, the patient must have real confidence in the physician, so that he can fully trust that he or she is receiving carefully thought out, individualized care from a knowledgeable expert. Second, the treatment itself should be logical and comprehensible in its technical aspects, side effects, and goals. At all times the patient should remember that the enemy is the cancer, and not the therapy (nor the physician).

One cannot generalize about chemotherapy, anymore than one can generalize about cancer. There are more than forty different drugs used, as well as multiple possible combinations. Each one is quite different, with side effects ranging from minimal to severe. As an example, most of the drugs do not cause significant hair loss, something that is strongly associated in many people's minds with chemotherapy. Focus only on the specifics of the program being recommended for you. It is important to grasp the difference between the two major ways chemotherapy is utilized. One of these is called "adjuvant chemotherapy"—the use of chemotherapy after initial surgery or radiation therapy, in an effort to treat possible microscopic residual disease, in order to prevent recurrence; this is often done, for example, in breast cancer. Adjuvant therapy is preventative, and there is no disease to measure or follow, so that there is no specific way to know "if it is working." The second use of chemotherapy is in the treatment of known recurrent cancer, in an effort to get the patient into remission, or cure the patient.

Try to develop an attitude about the therapy that enables you best to work with it and tolerate the treatment. An example of "attitude adjustment" might be the following: A common adjuvant program for breast cancer consists of eight treatments given every three weeks, requiring six months to complete. Rather than thinking of it as six months of chemotherapy, think of it instead as eight days of chemotherapy, spread out over six months. As much as possible, fit the chemotherapy into your life, rather than wrapping your life around chemotherapy.

Feel free to ask about possible alternatives to the proposed treatment, and strive for a clear sense why such alternatives are thought not to be as beneficial as the recommended treatment. It may well be necessary to obtain other opinions in order to develop the needed level of confidence in the plan. If the physician cannot understand the need for such opinions, change doctors. However, be aware that there is a great deal of valid disagreement amongst oncologists, based on personal experience and their own interpretation of the published literature. It's very possible to get a differing, yet reasonable, opinion that will have to be reconciled with the first opinion.

At all times, try to take the long view, keeping your thoughts and concentration on the horizon of long-term goals, rather than on the immediate individual steps required to get there. Cancer is a challenge, not only to your physical tolerance of discomfort and inconvenience, but, even more so, to your emotional stability and spiritual strength. Those who are able to extract some positive value from the experience seem to cope the best with these challenges. Of course, no one wants to develop cancer, but, if it does happen to you, try to use it in some way to learn to love and respect yourself more—even viewing it as a possible turning point in your life. Have your goal go beyond trying to beat your cancer or simply live as well and as long as you can with it: Gain from the experience positive personal revelations of lasting value.

As you undergo chemotherapy (or any therapy), it might be helpful to keep the following in mind:

- Focus on the purpose of the therapy, and what it can accomplish for you, rather than on the negative (the "side effects").
- Understand the likely and predictable problems you might have to endure with your therapy. Do not be concerned with anything you might have heard generally about chemotherapy, or about someone else's experience with chemotherapy.
- Take the long view and see the positive benefits as lasting. Chemotherapy is often a short-term investment for a long-term gain.
- Understand that the chemotherapy and you form the team against the enemy, the cancer. Do not fall into the trap of seeing treatment as the element to be resisted.

- Gather enough information and understanding to be confident that the treatment is the right one for you. At that point, the treatment becomes your ally, something you can work with and not something "being done to you." If you adopt a healthy attitude, the chemotherapy will feel less like a violation to your physical body and mental health.

- Do not be hesitant to turn to those around you for support and help. As helpful and comforting to you as this will be, it will be very rewarding and gratifying to your family and friends to be able to assist you. Give them that opportunity, and embrace their support.

As you begin this book, make a commitment to yourself that you are going to do all in your power in your personal battle with cancer. Your weapons include not only the advances made by medical science, but also those attitudes and hopes that you bring to the situation. This book will become a real asset in the development of your understanding of chemotherapy, which can be your potent ally. Now, go forward into your treatment with understanding, optimism, and energy.

Michael B. Van Scoy-Mosher, M.D., M.A.

Dr. Michael B. Van Scoy-Mosher graduated from the Albert Einstein School of Medicine in New York in 1966 and received advanced training in medical oncology at the Yale University School of Medicine and at the National Institute of Health. With a master's degree from the University of Southern California's Annenberg School of Communication and a continuing interest in health education, Dr. Van Scoy-Mosher has contributed to many print and video communications projects including the National Cancer Institute's publication, "Chemotherapy and You," and the award-winning film Destined to Live. *Dr. Van Scoy-Mosher is currently an attending oncologist at Cedars-Sinai Medical Center in Los Angeles, where he chairs the bioethics committee and the breast cancer tumor board.*

1

CHEMOTHERAPY TODAY

CANCER CURE RATES HAVE DRAMATICALLY IMPROVED

AS YOU BEGIN THIS BOOK, YOU MAY NOT HAVE BEGUN CHEMOTHERAPY treatments. Or you might feel you need help to fight your way through to the end of your treatment for cancer, which may be many months away. You or your family may fear the unknown physical and emotional shocks that lie ahead. You may be grappling to discover just exactly what life will hold when chemotherapy is finally complete, and you're ready to move on.

Unfortunately, it is still commonly believed that chemotherapy offers no real hope of curing cancer. Exactly the opposite is true. Chemotherapy is the most rapidly changing and dynamic area of modern cancer treatment, and breakthroughs in new chemotherapy drugs and treatment techniques continue to occur.

The good news is that chemotherapy treatment has become quite sophisticated. Many, many thousands of people receive chemotherapy today, and many find that their treatments result in fewer and milder side effects than they imagined. New anticancer drugs, new antinausea and pain medications, and new medical technology have created a more comfortable and efficient healing environment. Practical new stress-relieving techniques and new holistic treatment strategies have made the physical and emotional side effects of chemotherapy less disruptive to most people's lives than ever before.

As you read this book, you may be surprised to learn that a great many people have only minor side effects from chemotherapy. Many people don't lose weight, and not everyone loses all his or her hair.

That said, it is important to note that, like many medical treatments, chemotherapy has not attained absolute perfection. You still might have serious side effects, and you might well experience significant emotional and social stress before your treatment program is over.

This book provides you with information to make your chemotherapy treatments more manageable. Included are practical suggestions to help you through the whole complex of problems you may encounter, including the physical, social, psychological, and even spiritual repercussions of chemotherapy. At the very least, reading this book gives you a foundation of knowledge with which to discuss your treatment with your medical team. And certainly in medical treatment, as in life, a bit of knowledge properly applied can alleviate a great deal of pain and suffering.

As health writer Norman Cousins has dramatically demonstrated, many patients have begun taking a more active role in their own treatment. This trend toward becoming a partner with your doctor is healthy. Many medical doctors believe that a more knowledgeable patient is ultimately a better patient. Research has shown that people who are educated about their disease and its treatment not only are better able to manage their symptoms, they may actually live longer with significantly higher quality lives.

Chemotherapy Today

Every year more than 200,000 people benefit from chemotherapy, according to the New York–based Chemotherapy Foundation. Mammoth new computer databases such as Physicians' Data Query (PDQ), available free through the National Cancer Institute, can instantaneously provide the most recent cancer treatment and research trial information to any doctor in the

United States. Medical information is increasingly available to the general public through PDQ as well as other on-line databases such as the National Library of Medicine's Cancerlit. In rural areas, new techniques such as telemedicine are making the expertise of top cancer specialists more available and accessible. Along the information superhighway, ad hoc discussion groups are forming that simply didn't exist a few years ago, bringing consumers many new possibilities for gathering and sharing information. Although the amount of medical knowledge grows by leaps and bounds, that knowledge is more readily available to the cancer patient today than ever before.

The Holistic Approach

In previous centuries, physicians had a much more "whole person" approach to illness than has medicine in the twentieth century. Many years ago, what the patient *said* was the primary tool a physician had to identify an illness, and the patient often participated in the healing process, however imperfect the medical treatment may have been. According to some medical historians, the invention of antiseptic and anesthesia at the turn of the century allowed for successful treatment of disease by purely medical interventions, such as surgery. By the early and mid-twentieth century, most doctors were focused on the physical treatment of a particular disease—on healing the body—which was natural enough since this was where the great medical successes were occurring. Quite innocently, factors such as the patient's emotional state and his or her quality of life may have been brushed aside as irrelevant.

These days, in good cancer care and many other branches of medicine such as pediatrics, the thinking has evolved back to include the healing of the whole patient, a stance generally known as holistic medicine, because it involves the whole person.

All the major comprehensive cancer research centers in the United States now utilize a multidisciplinary approach to treating cancer. As the term implies, the multidisciplinary approach used at all the nation's best cancer care centers includes not only good medical treatment, but a strategy for healing that also involves the patient with other disciplines such as psychology, education, and nutrition. The multidisciplinary approach can involve new techniques or strategies such as visual imaging, and support groups that can address a patient's important psychosocial needs.

Inside and outside the research hospital, a growing body of scientific research supports this new holistic approach to medical care. Some of the pressure for change has admittedly come up from the grassroots, because of people who are not medical doctors such as Norman Cousins and Harold Benjamin. Within the boundaries of good medical practice, the holistic approach seeks to involve both the patient's mind and the patient's body in the healing process. The holistic approach to cancer treatment is the approach taken in this book, because it includes all the proven tools and techniques available today, and encourages you to put all those tools into the service of your recovery.

Long History

The vivid and gruesome details of hard-drinking, cigar-smoking General Ulysses S. Grant's battle against throat cancer captivated the nation a hundred years ago. In Victorian times, doctors believed that "cancer equals death." It was common practice for doctors not to even tell their patients they had cancer, because curing cancer was considered impossible.

Many famous people, such as Sigmund Freud, George Gershwin, Eva Peron, Rachel Carson, Duke Ellington, Babe Ruth, Mickey Mantle, Adelle Davis, and Humphrey Bogart were diagnosed with cancer. Novelist Alexander Solzhenitsyn, actress Shirley Temple Black, prime minister Golda Meir, and opera singer Beverly Sills are among the many people who fought cancer and survived, living active and productive lives for many years after good medical care drove their cancer into remission. Western movie star John Wayne died a well-publicized death from lung cancer, but his cancer was kept in remission for more than seven years by good medical treatment.

President Lyndon Johnson survived skin cancer. President

Ronald Reagan survived colon cancer after it was discovered in the summer of 1985.

Richard Block, a co-founder of the tax firm H&R Block, was advised by a physician to "get your estate in order" when he was diagnosed with terminal lung cancer in 1978. Instead, Block found other doctors and put himself through an aggressive course of surgery, radiation, immunotherapy, and chemotherapy on his way to being cured of lung cancer. According to author Judith Glassman, Block was undergoing chemotherapy when he quipped, "If these drugs could make this big, strong body so violently ill, think what they would be doing to these weak little cancer cells." After he recovered, Block was a prime mover in creating the PDQ database, the first and most comprehensive such data bank of cancer treatments in the world.

Positive Outlook

Bernie Siegel, M.D., is a Yale University cancer surgeon who has written several inspirational books about the psychological and social, or psychosocial, aspects of cancer. A cancer patient beginning treatment once asked Dr. Siegel if he could get well.

"Of course you can," Dr. Siegel replied. "Statistics may be against you, but there's no reason you can't get well."

Dr. Siegel later noted that the fact that one person recovered from a particular disease gave him—and the patient—the right to assume that another person might recover, too. Without creating any false hope, Dr. Siegel believes that he has the right to suggest that any person undergoing treatment might well be the first person to survive a particular cancer. As he has often observed, no one ever died of statistics.

Leaps and Bounds

According to the American Cancer Society, only about 20 percent of cancer patients could expect to be cured of cancer in 1925. By 1955 survival rates had increased to about 33 percent. By 1976 survival rates increased to about 41 percent, reflecting more effective use of surgery, radiation therapy, and new techniques such as chemotherapy than ever before.

Survival rates continue to rise as doctors and patients learn more about treating and preventing cancer.

According to the National Cancer Institute's 1994 statistical review, nearly 54 percent of all people of all ages who developed any kind of malignant growth between 1983 and 1990 could expect to be "cured," that is, to survive at least five years after their treatment for cancer. For people under sixty-five years of age, the overall five-year survival rate was almost 58 percent.

For skin cancer or *in situ* cancer of the cervix, survival rates now approach 100 percent. When all age groups are considered, five-year survival rates for people diagnosed at every stage of thyroid and testes cancer are now more than 90 percent. Five-year survival rates for melanoma, corpus uteri, and breast cancer are more than 80 percent. Urinary bladder cancer and Hodgkin's disease survival rates exceed 75 percent even when the most advanced cases are included. Survival rates for childhood leukemia have improved from about 20 percent in the late 1970s to more than 60 percent today.

Since cancer treatment continues to improve, if you were diagnosed with cancer this year, your chances of surviving cancer are probably even better than the published statistics indicate, since it takes a lag of at least five years to even calculate mortality.

Chemotherapy has already had an important role in bringing survival rates up and cancer mortality down in several types of cancer including lymphatic leukemia, lymphoma, some sarcomas, Hodgkin's disease, choriocarcinoma, and breast, bone, and testicular cancer. Promising results are being obtained from the use of chemotherapy in treating ovarian and colon cancers, and some lung and gastrointestinal cancers are beginning to show a response to chemotherapy.

Today, the average patient with cancer lives longer than the average person who suffers a severe heart attack. Interestingly enough, the National Cancer Institute estimates that cancer mortality would drop an *additional* 10 percent if the latest treatment methods were used on every person diagnosed with cancer today.

That millions of people regularly survive a once incurable disease like cancer is an unacknowledged miracle of modern medicine.

Overview

This book is designed to give you and perhaps your family and friends a working knowledge of chemotherapy as a treatment for cancer, emphasizing the many ways in which patients may take positive action to participate in their own treatment and recovery. It includes case histories of people who have been cured of cancer with chemotherapy. The first section of this book focuses on the medical aspects of chemotherapy, while the second section deals with the many other important aspects of cancer treatment.

Chapter 2 provides an overview of cancer, and chapter 3 describes the ways in which chemotherapy is employed in its treatment today. Chapter 4 lists some of the most common misconceptions about chemotherapy and cancer in a question-and-answer format that provides accurate information with which to combat these stubborn myths.

Chapter 5 explains how doctors arrive at a recommendation for chemotherapy, including the types of risks and benefits they consider. Chapter 6 discusses where you might wish to receive chemotherapy treatment, and includes an explanation and discussion of clinical research trials.

Chapter 7 provides an overview of your cancer treatment team, including medical specialists and other professionals you may expect to encounter during your chemotherapy treatment. It includes a quick checklist of things you might want to do before beginning chemotherapy treatments. Chapter 8 discusses the ways in which chemotherapy treatments may be administered. Chapter 9 explains why it is important to be an educated patient, and includes suggestions for effectively communicating with your medical team.

Chapter 10 provides a comprehensive list of the fifty-seven most commonly used anticancer drugs, including information on the types of cancer for which particular drugs are used, and their most common side effects.

Chapter 11 lists many of the most common physical side effects of chemotherapy, and includes tips on dealing with them.

Chapter 12 deals with the potentially healing effects of good nutrition, an area of interest to many people. Chapter 13 contains tips on maintaining your physical appearance during chemotherapy, including some health tips. Chapter 14 deals with the most common complaint of cancer patients—physical pain—and discusses how and why any pain you experience might be alleviated.

Chapter 15 discusses the debilitating issue of emotional stress, and offers some tips on maintaining a positive attitude during treatment. Chapter 16 lists proven alternative techniques and methods you may use to relieve your own psychological stress and relieve physical pain. Chapter 17 discusses the ways you may get help from the people around you, including the people in your life, and new people you might meet such as those in support groups, as well as spiritual issues often encountered during treatment that can sometimes result in a very happy ending.

Chapter 18 examines the financial aspects of chemotherapy treatment, including tips on dealing with health insurance companies, and some possible sources of financial help for all people.

Chapter 19 looks at unproven or unorthodox cancer therapy treatments, explains why they are popular, and suggests how they may sometimes be coordinated with basic good medical care provided by your doctor.

Chapter 20 focuses on the process of getting your life back in order after chemotherapy treatments are completed, including the common concerns and fears that many people experience once their treatments for cancer are completed.

Chapter 21 includes some thoughts to consider if your chemotherapy doesn't work.

Appendices to this book include New Treatments, discussing some new treatment strategies on the horizon. A very useful and practical Other Resources appendix lists toll-free phone numbers and addresses for major cancer organizations that provide additional information, as well as Internet addresses, and a short reading list of other books. A Glossary of Common Terms appendix is included to help you understand some of the unfamiliar words you might encounter over the next several months.

Freight Train

Being told you have cancer probably hit you like a freight train. Receiving an unwanted diagnosis of cancer has surely churned up a lot of powerful emotions in you such as rage, sadness, fear, even depression. You may feel quite confused. Your work life, your social life, even your family life may be already perilously disrupted. If you are among the 1 million Americans diagnosed with cancer this year, you may be stuck in the process of grieving for the healthy freedom of the life you feel you have lost, and wondering if your body or your personal life will ever be the same again now that you are entering uncharted waters.

Since dread of the unknown is for many people worse than the actual experience, this book will help you arm yourself with information in your personal battle against cancer. Take heart in knowing that your personal battle is more winnable than ever before in the history of medicine.

The information contained in this book may not solve all the problems in your life, but it will help you make your chemotherapy treatments more manageable.

Everyone doesn't survive cancer. But almost everyone survives chemotherapy, which typically lasts between three months and three years.

Remember that the enemy is not chemotherapy. The enemy is cancer.

By passing through several months of chemotherapy, and taking good care of yourself as you heal, you may considerably lengthen and improve the quality of your own life.

PART I

MEDICAL ASPECTS OF CHEMOTHERAPY

Healing is a matter of time,
but it is sometimes also a matter of opportunity.
HIPPOCRATES

2

ABOUT CANCER

HOW CANCER DEVELOPS AND SPREADS

ALTHOUGH WE DON'T YET FULLY UNDERSTAND THE BIOLOGY OF cancer, medical science already knows how to drive it into remission most of the time. This chapter describes how cancer begins inside your body, develops, spreads, and is identified prior to treatment. Comprehending cancer will help you understand how medical treatment can control it.

If you are like a lot of people, you already know cancer is serious. You may have encountered bits of information in magazine articles or on television newscasts, but these fragments of information probably don't add up to a clear picture of this mysterious disease.

Think of cancer as a nest of termites inside your sturdy old wooden farmhouse. The termites don't appear to be a problem at first. In fact, you probably don't even know you *have* termites for a long time. But termites cause problems if they multiply and spread, because they eat away roof support beams, which eventually will bring your wooden house crashing to the ground. Remember that termites can't destroy your house if you discover them early and get your house fumigated, which is what chemotherapy can do to cancer.

Dealing with cancer isn't easy. Modern medicine works miracles, but receiving medical treatment may make you feel as if you've been swept onto the set of a science fiction movie like *Star*

Wars. You may feel small, powerless, and confused as you trek into a universe of pungent medicinal smells, where medical people come and go in smocks, rubber gloves, and face masks, exchanging medical terms you don't understand. Understand that this book will demystify your medical treatment—whose purpose, after all, is only to help you. It's all right to feel apprehensive. Just understand that the next few months will be easier and less threatening if you take steps to educate and help yourself.

A lot of people get cancer. Health organizations estimate that one in every three persons now alive will be diagnosed with cancer in their lifetime. No group is immune. Corporate titans, star athletes, health nuts, homemakers, and couch potatoes . . . people from every walk of life are treated for cancer. One reason that incidences of cancer are rising has to do with the very success of modern medicine, which has conquered many previously fatal diseases like polio, tuberculosis, and smallpox, thus allowing us all to live the longer lives that also allow for an increased chance of developing cancer. Unfortunately, incidences of cancer do become more frequent as people age. The American Cancer Society estimates that 60 percent of all cancers occur in people over the age of sixty-five, and incidences are higher in the highest age groups. Nonetheless, a few types of cancers, such as testicular cancer or Hodgkin's disease, are far more likely to occur in children or young people.

Cancer is an old disease. References to cancer may be found in the writings of ancient Egyptians. The word itself can be traced to the writings of Hippocrates. In the fifth century B.C., more than two thousand years ago, Hippocrates applied the Greek word for crab, *karkinoma,* to the long and distended veins extending out from untreated breast cancers, which he apparently thought resembled the extended claws of a crab. The Latin word for crab, *cancer,* is still used today.

Cancer Takes Many Forms

Cancer is actually a generic term for a group of about two hundred similar but distinctive diseases that all advance and spread in slightly different ways. This includes more than twenty identified types of leukemia, which are all cancers of the white blood cells but with different characteristics. Some cancers progress slowly, and some rapidly. One fairly common type of cancer, prostate cancer, grows so slowly that a lot of men live to a happy old age and die without ever realizing that they had it. In one rare type of childhood cancer, Burkitt's lymphoma, tumors have been known to grow so quickly that they almost double in size in forty-eight hours.

Unlike most diseases, cancer does not occur because your body is exposed to an outside bacteria, a fungus, or a virus. Cancer begins within the cells of your own body, in an elusive biochemical process that is still not fully understood by medical professionals.

A Rogue Cell

Microbiologists think every person's body creates cancerous cells, even people who never get cancer. Indeed, most people may produce several cancerous cells every day. But under normal circumstances, these rogue cells are destroyed by your white blood cells, the front line of your body's immune system. Your immune system normally intercepts and kills these stray mutant cancer cells before they can multiply and grow into what we think of as cancer.

All types of cancer are characterized by the creation of wild, mutant living cells whose growth cannot be restricted to a single location. The current thinking is that a normal cell takes a series of biological "hits," causing it to become cancerous. This one mutating cancer cell loses its biological discipline and begins dividing much more quickly than normal and much earlier than normal. It produces lots of unusual looking cell offspring, which don't function as normal cells but which keep reproducing anyway. The place where cancer begins is known as the *primary site*.

Cancer cells divide and divide again, a process that can take several years. At some point, cancer cells may break off from the malignant tumor, drift through the bloodstream, and try to start tiny new cancer colonies in other parts of the body. Most of the

15

time, it is this spread of cancer cells that makes cancer dangerous to your health.

Any mass of cells without a biological purpose in the body can be called a tumor. A *benign tumor* doesn't really spread, so it is harmless. A *malignant tumor* is a mass of cells that is cancerous, and because malignant tumors spread, they are not harmless at all.

Malignant tumors are not harmful in themselves. The physical danger comes when a cancer colony spreads, growing into or attaching itself to a major organ such as the kidney, heart, or brain. If cancer is not stopped, it will grow into your organ's vital tissues, disable the organ's normal function, and indirectly cause your death.

Cancer spreads or *metastasizes* quickly or slowly, depending on the type of cancer, but is usually painless in the early stages. By the time a tumor can be detected by a medical doctor, it has grown to approximately one-half inch in diameter and contains nearly a *billion* cells. At this point, the original cell has already doubled about thirty times.

Cancer is a disease of the human body, not of the soul. It is important for you to realize that cancer is not a punishment for past sins, any more than is a case of the measles. Today, doctors look at cancer as a set of chronic diseases that can frequently be medically controlled, somewhat similar to high blood pressure or diabetes. Due to treatments such as chemotherapy that can control or eliminate cancer, the average cancer patient already lives longer than the average patient who has heart trouble.

Identifying Cancer

Cancer that begins in an organ is diagnosed or named according to where it originates in the body, if this can be determined. If the cancer's primary site is in the lungs, for example, the cancer cells will almost always look like mutant lung cells under the microscope even if the cancer has spread to another part of the body. Since this cancer began in the lungs, it is always called lung cancer. If it began in the breast, it would be called breast cancer, and so on.

The basic types of cancers include *carcinoma,* cancer that originates in the lining or covering tissues of ducts or organs, which is
by far the most common type of cancer. A *sarcoma* is a cancer of
soft tissues that begins in the muscles, nerves, tendons, blood ves-
sels, or bones. *Lymphoma* is a cancer that begins in the lymph system. *Leukemia* is a cancer that begins in the white blood cells. A
multiple myeloma is cancer that begins in the plasma cells within
the bone marrow.

It is important that your physician identifies the biology of
your cancer as soon as possible, because he or she can use this information to predict the cancer's behavior. In addition to a minor
surgical operation called a *biopsy*, you may expect to get a few
tests and lab work done before your cancer is identified. By a
process of logic and deduction, identifying the biology of the cancer and its stage of growth will help your doctor present the best
available treatment options to you.

Cancer is actually a group of similar diseases, which all begin
inside the human body. Fortunately, you have only one type of
cancer with which to contend, and that cancer may be treatable.
The next chapter explains the important role that chemotherapy
can play in the treatment of your disease.

3

ABOUT CHEMOTHERAPY

How Chemotherapy Is Used to Treat Cancer

CHEMOTHERAPY BASICALLY MEANS MEDICAL TREATMENT WITH CHEMICALS, and it has become one of the primary methods of treating cancer. This chapter explains how doctors use chemotherapy in combination with other treatments, how chemotherapy works, and why combinations of chemotherapy drugs can be effective.

Remember that 8 million Americans are alive today who have been diagnosed with cancer, including 4 million diagnosed within the past five years. Sophisticated medical treatment is the reason why most of these people are expected to survive and live normal life spans.

The three basic treatments for cancer are surgery, radiation therapy, and chemotherapy. These three treatment *modalities* have cured thousands and thousands of cases of cancer, relieved much pain and suffering, and extended many lives far beyond what could have been reasonably expected if the cancer was left untreated.

The three treatments may be used separately, but they are often used in tandem to treat particular types of cancer, a strategy known as *multimodality* therapy. A fourth well-publicized but still primarily investigational treatment is *immunotherapy*, which involves the use of purified proteins such as interferon and interleukin-2 to strengthen the immune system. Immunotherapy is sometimes used together with chemotherapy, a treatment known as *chemoimmunotherapy*.

Chemotherapy is the newest of the three major cancer treatments, and it remains the most rapidly evolving area of cancer control. Chemotherapy treats cancer with "anticancer" drugs, agents or chemicals introduced into the body, either one at a time or in particular combinations. Although the rate of discovery for new anticancer agents has slowed, new drugs such as taxol, a natural substance made from the bark of the Pacific yew tree, continue to be approved. And research continues.

As many cancer survivors would quickly testify, chemotherapy can help save your life.

Peter's Story

A few days after he turned thirty, a big, athletic young man we shall call Peter saw a doctor because one of his testicles was swollen. He was diagnosed with testicular cancer, one of the most rapidly growing of all cancers. Peter's cancer was stage B-3, meaning it had already spread up the left side of his body through his lymph nodes.

Within a few days, Peter had surgery to have the testicle removed. After that, he received several months of chemotherapy to shrink the metastasized cancer before it was surgically removed in a second operation, at a comprehensive cancer center in the Northwest. Peter's multimodality treatment for cancer cost $70,000, but fortunately his health insurance paid all but $75 of the costs.

"Testicular cancer grows very fast. By going in early and receiving treatment, I probably saved my life," Peter says today. "A lot of guys go into denial when they are diagnosed, and don't get treatment until it's too late."

When presented with the treatment options by his medical oncologist, Peter quickly agreed to a very aggressive course of treatment, which also has a very high rate of success. He received combination chemotherapy with a "PEB" regimen consisting of three chemotherapy drugs—cisplatin, etoposide, and bleomycin.

Peter received chemotherapy for a week in the hospital, and then had three weeks off to recover before the next cycle of chemotherapy began.

A "go for broke" race car driver and scuba diver, Peter kept a nonchalantly positive attitude all the way through his year-long ordeal. He focused his energy on getting well. He never lost his sense of humor. He was amused when the nurse who was giving him chemotherapy spilled a drop of the chemotherapy drug on her finger, and immediately dropped everything she was doing to run over to the sink and wash her hands. Peter laughed when he realized that the material being injected into his body was something a nurse was frightened to spatter on her finger—and he ribbed her about it.

Even though he was fairly young, Peter had led an active, risk-taking life. "The danger to my life never seemed very immediate," Peter says of medical treatment. "I tried to keep a positive attitude. My aim was to just get through it. I wanted to get out of that place."

Peter felt fine during the first round of chemotherapy, but when the second cycle began he suffered side effects of queasiness, cold sores, lethargy, and loss of hair. "By the third day of my second cycle I'd really get hit. You knew they were pumping poison into you," Peter recalled.

In the weeks between Peter's last three chemotherapy treatments, all six feet, 2 inches of his body felt weak and lethargic. He was unable to work. He spent time at home reading books, cooking good meals for himself, and doing something he'd never done before—watching an entire World Series. His doctor complimented him on his high blood counts and fast healing, and was quite surprised to see that Peter actually gained weight beyond his normal 220 pounds.

Peter's roommate was frightened and withdrew during Peter's medical treatment. But Peter's father, stepmother, and two brothers supported him by frequently visiting when he was in the hospital.

"But I just hated people standing at the end of my hospital bed looking at me with that doleful look," Peter recalls. He admits that sometimes the expressions on the faces of his visitors—even his own father—made him angry enough to shout. Peter learned that hospital rooms have clocks with seconds hands to remind patients that time is passing.

After chemotherapy, Peter underwent an eight-and-a-half hour operation to remove what he saw as the enemy—"the monster inside me"—the cancer that had spread. There were some complications from the long surgery, but it was successful and all the cancer was removed.

Two years is the period of greatest concern for testicular cancer, a time when more than 90 percent of the recurrences appear. For two years, Peter got a blood test every three months and a CAT scan every six months. All those tests showed his cancer was firmly in remission. That was four years ago.

Although he walked with a cane for a few months after surgery, Peter has recently begun jogging again and educating himself for a new career.

"People need to keep a positive mental attitude, and to understand that medical treatment doesn't last forever. Do whatever you have to do to get through it," Peter advises. "Know you're going to get sick, but you're going to get better, too."

Chemotherapy Drugs

Several dozen chemotherapy drugs have been approved for use either singly or in combination with other drugs by the U.S. Food and Drug Administration. Anticancer drugs may be taken as pills, injected into the body, or a few applied as skin patches and allowed to soak into the skin. Very occasionally, anticancer drugs can be pumped directly into an organ such as the liver through a connecting artery, or injected directly into the abdominal cavity. Very rarely, as in some cases of Kaposi's sarcoma, diluted solutions of chemotherapy drugs such as vinblastine are injected directly into skin lesions as a way of treating the tumor.

Chemotherapy is broadly different from surgery or radiation therapy, both in the way it is delivered and in its ultimate effects.

Chemotherapy is almost always systemic, that is, the chemicals used to kill cancer cells circulate throughout your body. This can create side effects, but it is also chemotherapy's greatest strength as a treatment. Because chemotherapy is systemic, it does not attack only tumors that have been detected. Chemotherapy can also seek out and kill tiny, undetectable colonies of cancer cells that may have broken off from the main tumor and drifted to other locations.

The ability to clean out every small, nearly invisible colony of cancer cells that exists in your body is the reason why chemotherapy is often the treatment of choice. This is why chemotherapy is given after surgery in many cases of breast cancer—treatment that has prevented thousands of recurrences of cancer.

Kills Invisible Tumors

Chemotherapy is used to kill small, nearly invisible tumors. Chemotherapy is used to shrink larger tumors prior to surgery or radiation treatment. Chemotherapy is used after surgery or radiation to mop up the remaining cancer cells that may have spread to other locations.

Chemotherapy is generally most effective on fast-growing cancers whose cells divide and reproduce very rapidly. For several cancers, chemotherapy is the treatment of choice. It is least effective on slow-growing cancers such as prostate cancer, which is why other treatments such as surgery and radiation are more frequently selected.

To achieve maximum effectiveness, chemotherapy is almost always administered in cycles. You may expect a period of receiving chemotherapy drugs to alternate with a rest period, in which your body recovers its strength. Receiving chemotherapy may be unlike any experience you have ever had before—for either medical or psychological reasons. But remember that educating yourself will give you a measure of control over many of chemotherapy's effects.

"At the first injection you are completely entering into the unknown," says a woman we shall call Selma, a program administrator who was cured of breast cancer by chemotherapy at the age of twenty-eight. "There's a whole aspect of being diagnosed with cancer, where you feel like your body becomes a clinical mechanism. When I started chemotherapy I truly felt out of control. It helped me a lot when I reminded myself that I chose chemotherapy, and that I was in control of that. It helped me to see that chemotherapy was something done *with* me, and not *to* me. Chemotherapy is systemic, that is, it involves the whole body. Chemotherapy is poison, but you have to take the poison to kill the disease."

Accidental Discovery

When a ship full of American sailors carrying deadly mustard gas exploded during World War II, pathologists were amazed by the damage to the lymph systems and bone marrow of the sailors who had died. After the war, physicians at Yale University experimented with a related gas, nitrogen mustard, to treat cancers of the blood and lymph system. These doctors were delighted to find that the treatment markedly (but temporarily) reduced the size of tumors. Thus, chemotherapy was born. Over the years, more than a quarter of a million different drugs have been tested in government-sponsored testing programs.

Cancer Specialists

Your family doctor or general practitioner should not attempt to treat cancer, which is normally handled by medical specialists. These days, cancer is usually treated by a very sophisticated medical team of *oncologists*, doctors who specialize in the treatment of cancer, including *medical oncologists* who normally recommend and plan chemotherapy treatment. Chapter 7 discusses the medical specialists you're likely to meet in greater detail.

Medical expertise in the field of chemotherapy is absolutely crucial, because most anticancer drugs are so toxic and powerful that other doctors typically don't prescribe them. With most chemotherapy agents, only a very fine line separates a therapeutic from a toxic dose. The margin between an effective dose of any chemotherapy drug and a fatal dose is called the *therapeutic index*. Of course, the doses you receive must be carefully calculated, and your reactions to chemotherapy monitored to achieve the best results.

Receiving Chemotherapy

You may receive chemotherapy treatments in a hospital room as an *inpatient,* or as an *outpatient* who comes to the hospital for treatments but doesn't spend the night. You may receive chemotherapy in a private doctor's office, a clinic, or sometimes even in your home. In all cases, the anticancer drugs you receive will be chosen by your doctor. Before you receive chemotherapy, you must understand its risks and benefits, and then agree to treatment by your doctor.

Your first round of chemotherapy is called first line chemotherapy, and this does the job for most people. If first line chemotherapy isn't effective, second line chemotherapy with another anticancer drug or drug combination is an option you and your doctor may consider.

The chemotherapy drugs currently approved for the treatment of cancer destroy cancer cells in different ways, that is, at different phases in their growth cycle. Most of them shake up the DNA of cancer cells. A listing of the major drug groups as well as the fifty-seven most commonly used anticancer drugs and their most common physical side effects may be found in chapter 10.

Combination Chemotherapy

As you have seen, a malignant tumor contains millions of cells, all constantly growing and dividing. Not all these cells are at the same stage of the growth cycle at any one time.

Most frequently, your medical oncologist will choose some combination of between two and twelve drugs to be given either in sequence, or concurrently during treatment. Using several anti-cancer agents simultaneously is called *combination chemotherapy*. From the universe of chemotherapy drugs, your medical oncologist may select only one drug to use in *single agent chemotherapy*, a treatment that works best on certain types of cancers such as some chronic leukemias. Ultimately the selection of chemotherapy drugs depends on the type of cancer, the stage of the cancer, and many other factors, including the patient's age and health.

Successes with combination chemotherapy began to occur during the 1960s. These days, thanks to thousands of clinical trials and a lot of medical research, combination chemotherapy has become quite sophisticated. Combinations of anticancer drugs pack a powerful wallop because they attack the growing and dividing cancer cells at several different stages of their growth cycle.

Combination chemotherapy can include drugs that help other anticancer drugs act more efficiently, or even drugs that mitigate the side effects of other drugs. For instance, stage B ovarian cancer might be treated with cycles of the so-called CHAP regimen of cisplatin or carboplatin in combination with Cytoxan, Adriamycin (doxorubicin), and hexamethylmelamine, or carboplatin and taxol. Colon cancer might be treated with surgery plus cycles of adjuvant chemotherapy using fluorouracil, but including leucovorin or levamisole to stimulate the immune system.

Hodgkin's disease might be treated with the four drug "MOPP" regimen comprised of mustargen, oncovin, prednisone, and procarbazine, which has pulled survival rates above 70 percent, even when statistics include patients in the most advanced stages, or with the newer "ABVD" combination chemotherapy of Adriamycin, bleomycin, vinblastine, and dacarbazine. These two accepted combination treatments for Hodgkin's disease may be used separately or in tandem to lessen the side effects of each set of drugs. *Crossover chemotherapy* is a more complex combination chemotherapy, where a second set of drugs is introduced to prevent resistance to a first set of drugs from developing, or to correct a poor response to the first chemotherapy.

Hormone therapy is frequently used in tandem with chemotherapy. As the name implies, hormone therapy involves treatment of cancer with hormones. Hormone therapy can be given prior to, instead of, or in addition to chemotherapy, but it works somewhat differently. For instance, breast cancers sometimes depend on particular female hormones for growth—in which case counterbalancing male hormones such as tamoxifen and androgen may be administered to block the growth of the breast cancer. Prostate cancer sometimes requires male hormones for growth, so a synthetic female hormone such as stilbestrol may be administered to block the production of male hormones, and slow the growth of the cancer.

Good Timing

Combinations of two or more anticancer drugs may be either administered simultaneously, or at intervals timed to hit the cancer cells at moments in their growth cycles when they are most vulnerable.

One advantage to you is that the anticancer drugs used in combination chemotherapy may be administered in lower doses than if the drugs were used alone. This results in less harm to your body and a faster recovery cycle. The use of drug combinations has even another advantage in that combinations can reduce your chances of developing resistance to a single drug, a development that occurs more frequently with single doses of higher potency.

Be reassured that a judicious and effective selection of anticancer drugs by your oncologist may result in fewer unpleasant side effects and a higher quality of life during and after your treatment for cancer.

Remember that the human body is tough and strong, and that cancer cells are not invincible. Very frequently, cancer cells are so weak and vulnerable that they die by the millions when exposed to chemotherapy drugs. Your body is a more complex organism than cancer, and you can help give yourself the strength to weather a chemical storm.

Properly administered chemotherapy helps people overcome cancer because chemotherapy is systemic. Chemotherapy drugs kill cancer cells. Drug combinations may be used to great effect. But before you are treated for cancer, or during your treatment, you may well encounter a few of the stubborn myths and misconceptions about cancer listed in the next chapter. Learning the truth will help you combat unhealthy attitudes you may encounter among your own family and friends—and help you in your personal battle for survival.

4

MYTHS AND MISCONCEPTIONS

SOME COMMON MYTHS ABOUT CANCER AND CHEMOTHERAPY

UNFORTUNATELY, MANY PEOPLE'S IDEAS ABOUT CHEMOTHERAPY, OR even cancer, are based on things they saw or overheard many years ago. Chemotherapy is a relatively new treatment for cancer, and much has changed in the years since chemotherapy was first employed for the treatment of cancer.

What follows is a list of some myths surrounding chemotherapy and cancer. Knowing the myths may help you recognize these attitudes in another person. Do you fear one of your friends is afraid they will "catch" cancer? Consider it your *duty* to set anyone straight if you hear one of these myths repeated. Speaking the truth will clear the air, and it may well make your life easier, too.

"Nobody ever survives chemotherapy, because chemotherapy is only given to people who are going to die."
Wrong. There is no medically accepted cancer treatment that doesn't produce survivors. Chemotherapy completely cures many people, and extends the life span of many more. While this may have often been true when chemotherapy was an experimental treatment, chemotherapy is now being successfully used earlier than ever before, such as before surgery or radiation to shrink can-

cer. Treatment methods are improved a bit every year and survival rates are climbing, meaning more people are living.

"Chemotherapy injections are very painful."
Wrong. Receiving chemotherapy treatments is painless, except for the rare cases when there is leakage of the anticancer medication out of the vein during treatment. Physical side effects, if they come at all, typically come hours or days afterward and are also frequently *not* painful.

"You always go bald when you get chemotherapy."
Maybe. Not every drug or combination of drugs causes hair loss, which is usually only temporary. The extent of hair loss varies quite a lot from person to person, and is not predictable. You can learn ways to minimize hair loss, as well as other side effects. Remember that even if you lose your hair, the hair almost always grows back—and sometimes thicker than before.

"Chemotherapy makes you sick."
Wrong. It's true that many chemotherapy drugs are quite toxic, but nausea can be effectively controlled in almost all chemotherapy patients, either through medication or through nonmedical methods such as relaxation techniques. With some anticancer drugs, nausea is never experienced at all.

"People taking chemotherapy get skinny as a rail."
Wrong. Many people actually gain a few pounds, particularly those on adjuvant chemotherapy, which is administered in rather small dosages. Much of the time, weight loss can be controlled through a combination of methods including simple changes in eating habits.

"You're a guinea pig when you get chemotherapy."
Wrong. All standard chemotherapy treatment protocols have been tested and approved, and many anticancer drugs have already been in use for several decades because they cure people. Only with your express written permission can you receive an experimental chemotherapy treatment in a clinical trial.

"If you don't get sick or have side effects, the chemotherapy isn't working."
Wrong. There is no relationship between toxic reactions to anti-cancer drugs and the suppression of cancer cells. For instance, some drugs have no side effects at all. Your doctor will give you tests that can measure the effectiveness of chemotherapy.

"If you get sick or have side effects, it means the cancer is coming back or getting stronger."
Wrong. There is no relationship between toxic reactions and the suppression of cancer cells. Different drugs produce different side effects in different people, and sometimes no side effects at all. Your doctor will give you tests that can measure the effectiveness of chemotherapy.

"People with cancer can't help themselves get well."
Wrong. There are many things patients can do to facilitate their own recoveries, such as assuring their own good nutrition and relaxing themselves with the stress-relieving and pain-relieving techniques touched upon in this book. Educating yourself about the procedures used to treat you, and things you need to do, can help you heal and improve the quality of your life.

"I did something wrong to make myself get cancer."
Incorrect. Having cancer is no more your own fault than if you come down with a common cold or break your arm. Cancer is a *medical* condition, not a divine punishment or self-fulfilling prophecy.

"My life is over since I've been diagnosed with cancer, because cancer is like a death sentence."
Wrong. Are you kidding? A lot of famous people such as former president Ronald Reagan have survived a bout or two with cancer and gone on to lead long and even more productive lives. The same is true for ordinary citizens. Remember, there are millions of cancer survivors living their lives quite productively at this very moment.

"You should be ashamed of getting cancer."
Wrong. It's not a mortal or even a venial sin to get sick. Cancer is a biological condition. Should you also be ashamed of contracting a common cold, getting the measles, or breaking your leg?

"Cancer is contagious."
No, no, no. This is one of the cruelest and most persistent myths of all. The fact is, no type of cancer is contagious in any way—not by touch, not by sneezing, not by kissing, not by sexual inter-course. Fear of contagion is a primitive and almost irrational fear, probably rooted in the instinct to survive, but it has no basis in fact when it comes to cancer. Cancer is *not* contagious. Cancer is *not* catching. Tell the world.

If you understand these and other medical misconceptions people may have about cancer or chemotherapy, it may well help you put your family and friends at ease. But as the next chapter explains, actually making the decision to have chemotherapy must be based on your doctor's recommendations—which spring from a definite set of medical facts.

5

THE CHEMOTHERAPY DECISION

HOW YOUR DOCTOR RECOMMENDS CHEMOTHERAPY

YOUR DECISION TO HAVE CHEMOTHERAPY COMES ONLY AT THE END of a kind of informational dance between you and your doctor. Your doctor must understand your health as well as the type and stage of your cancer before recommending treatment, which involves interpreting your test results. You must understand something about your disease and the risks and benefits of what chemotherapy can achieve before you approve your treatment plan. After this exchange of information, which can take a few days or a few weeks, the medical treatment can begin.

Ultimately the decision to undertake a particular regimen of chemotherapy treatments is yours.

After you have been diagnosed with cancer, but before you actually begin chemotherapy, your medical oncologist will present you with a range of treatment options, including the risks and benefits of each option. If your oncologist recommends a particular course of chemotherapy, you should clearly understand what the doctor hopes will be the end result of treatment.

In most cases you should seek another doctor's opinion before you decide to proceed with chemotherapy. Tell your doctor you wish to do this. Receiving a second opinion should give you more confidence in your doctor's diagnosis, and illuminate more clearly the path down which you should proceed.

Two Vows

Remember that chemotherapy is used against cancer because it works. But a number of variables factor into the probable success of chemotherapy, such as the age of the patient, the stage of the disease, and the types of anticancer agents chosen to treat the disease. It is important to remember that no two cases of cancer are exactly the same.

Oncologists can predict the direction in which your tumor might spread, but they cannot predict the speed at which it will move, which can be either faster or slower than most. Oncologists realize that different individuals can respond somewhat differently to chemotherapy, making cancer frustrating to treat.

Before you make the decision to begin chemotherapy, you should make two important vows to yourself:

1. I vow that I want to get well.
2. I vow that I will participate in my treatment even if it means enduring physical or emotional changes in my life.

Ideally, you will also resolve to educate yourself about ways to deal with chemotherapy's impact on you, and to take some action to help you control the process. As the following case history demonstrates, you *can* find your own way to handle the physical and psychosocial side effects you might encounter.

Krista's Story

A woman we shall call Krista was living in a remote mountainous area when, without warning, she was diagnosed with breast cancer at the age of forty-three. Married for nineteen years, trim, athletic Krista was the picture of good health. She had been running almost twenty miles a week for nearly as long as she had been married. She took vitamin supplements and thought of herself as an extremely healthy person. At first, she was shocked by her diagnosis.

"I was absolutely shocked that me, the healthiest person in our family, got cancer. I guess I believed the runner's myth—that you never get sick if you run," says Krista. "I felt angry, and I felt worthless. For me, cancer really was a wake-up call."

About a month after surgery removed the tumor from her breast, Krista began receiving combination chemotherapy treatments and radiation therapy.

Krista was finishing up a second round of combination chemotherapy at the time of this interview, when she was able to look back on the chaos of her previous year.

"It was a real shock to lose my hair and my breast at the same time. For a while I was just vegetating. I couldn't even cook a meal. I was mad at life, but I wanted to live," Krista says. "Looking back on it, I think I was living in the past and future, and dying in the present."

Krista lost her hair. During one chemotherapy treatment, the oncology nurse had to stick her five times to find a vein. Krista went through menopause, with hot flashes that made her body temperature shoot up five to seven degrees, several times a day. She complained about the hot flashes to her radiation oncologist and he said, "Just deal with it," a remark which struck her as cold and cruel.

Krista realized she wanted a divorce. As she received treatment for cancer, Krista fell into a depression that lasted four months. She even stopped the thing she loved the most—running. Her excuse was that the snow had begun to fall near her mountain home.

It took time and effort for Krista to pull herself out of the depression. She tried attending a support group, but it didn't work for her. She tried going back to church, but that didn't work either. She took antidepressant medication. She remembers once looking down at a pill she was taking and saying to herself, "If only I could run, I wouldn't have to take this pill."

Slowly, Krista worked her way out of the depression.

The turning point occurred shortly after she decided to visit a counselor's office at the comprehensive cancer center hospital where she was receiving treatment. The counselor listened. She reminded Krista of her own inner strength. When Krista left the office she remembers feeling "like a weight had been lifted off my shoulders . . . for some reason, hearing it from her was different than hearing it from family members or friends."

After notifying her doctor, she stopped her antidepressant medication. Her oncologist advised her to begin running again, and she did. Her doctor told her about a spring-loaded exercise device that would build up the walls of her veins, and she began exercises that made it easier for her to tolerate chemotherapy. Her life began to knit back together.

At the time of this interview, Krista had separated from her husband, and was making plans to move to another city. She had already worked her way up to running three to four miles at a time, in training for her first marathon race. She took up horseback riding again, one of the joys of her youth. "When I'm on that horse, I don't think about cancer. I feel like another person," Krista admits.

Krista got involved in a cancer fund-raising event, a run, and sent out sixty letters to her family and friends. As a result of her activity, she's proud to report she raised $1,660 mostly in $10 donations. She admits to feeling a great surge of accomplishment as she received and logged in each check.

Pleasantly, Krista has rediscovered her sense of humor. She has named her artificial breast "Kato," and she jokingly refers to herself as "Chemo Woman," a play on Wonder Woman. She eats nutritiously, drinking no coffee or tea, and takes five vitamin supplements a day as she has always done. She is delighted that her friends are positive, upbeat people and that her life seems back on track—at last.

"You do what you have to do to not go crazy," says Krista, who is planning to use her college degree in community health for the first time. "I know I feel like I'm back in control of my life. I'm just taking it one day at a time. I'm planning for the immediate future. I know I can't worry about what happened five years ago. The little things don't upset me anymore."

The Chemotherapy Decision

As Krista and many other people treated for cancer have learned, oncologists look at many factors before recommending a course of treatment, including the biology of the cancer and its stage of growth.

The biology of the cancer is of great importance. Cancer that begins in the breast will always act like breast cancer, even if it spreads to other parts of the body, so it's important to determine exactly which *type* of cancer you have, if that is possible. Since many types of cancer have fairly predictable patterns of growth, identifying the type of cancer helps your doctor plan a strategy to control it. In almost every case, a *biopsy* will be performed to remove a small sample of tumor tissue to be analyzed in the laboratory. The biopsy helps determine not only if you have cancer, but the particular type of cancer you have.

You'll receive more medical tests to determine the developmental status of your cancer, or which stage of growth it's in, a process called *staging*. The staging process typically involves taking a medical history, physical examinations, blood tests, and other tests such as x-rays and computed axial tomography (CAT) scans to first determine the size of the tumor, and then to look for evidence as to whether the tumor has spread to other sites in the body. Magnetic resonance imaging (MRI) is an imaging procedure that produces images of structures inside the body such as lymph nodes, bones, or the brain.

The more complex medical tests are frequently performed by medical technicians, sometimes in a medical laboratory at the hospital, or at another location. Your test results may be analyzed by a pathologist or another medical specialist, but the results return to the hands of your medical oncologist to help the doctor determine how far your cancer has spread. Accurately staging your cancer is quite important, because different stages of cancer respond differently to different treatments.

Since there are so many types of cancer, not everyone with cancer receives the same tests. Some types of cancer require specific tests to chart the progress, or lack of progress, of the disease. For instance, breast cancer patients receive mammograms, special x-ray tests that help detect tumors in the breast. Since prostate cancer frequently metastasizes to the bone, bone scans may be given to see whether the prostate cancer has spread. Cancer of the bowels frequently spreads to the liver, so liver scans and blood tests are used to determine whether or not the cancer has spread to those areas. Although the volume of tests can be time consuming and often emotionally taxing, they are necessary to your doctor in staging your disease.

Tumor Board

Before making treatment recommendations, your oncologist may consult informally with other medical specialists and share the results of your tests, x-rays, and other information. This may be done informally, as among the specialists at a particular clinic. A more formal way of doing this is to take the information in front of a hospital's tumor board, where specialists meet to discuss particular cases and offer treatment alternatives.

Patient identities are not revealed at tumor boards, but your pathologist might present the results of the biopsy, your radiologist the results of your x-rays, and so forth. The largest cancer treatment hospitals even have tumor boards that review particular types of cancer, such as tumor boards for breast cancer. This collaborative process can help your doctor get the best available ideas on the treatment alternatives. Ultimately, all this is formally presented to you, along with your doctor's recommendations.

Even if you live in a small town, this type of collaboration is starting to become available. A few rural hospitals and medical centers around the United States are employing the new technique of telemedicine as part of the process of recommending a treatment for cancer. Telemedicine allows doctors in smaller towns and smaller hospitals an opportunity to teleconference with oncologists in urban cancer treatment centers. With test results and other information sent along via computer modem for the experts to evaluate prior to the teleconference, telemedicine creates a virtual tumor board in cyberspace, which can be conducted as a video telephone conference between specialists hundreds of miles apart to determine a course of treatment on a particular patient.

Risks and Benefits

Potential risks and benefits are present in every treatment for cancer. When your oncologist formally presents treatment recommendations to you, your test results and the staging of your cancer should be explained, along with any information gathered from a tumor board or a review of the information by other physicians.

In recommending a course of chemotherapy, your oncologist must look at the big picture, including factors such as your age and the general state of your health. Age is a factor, for instance, because older people with weaker kidneys may not tolerate as aggressive a course of chemotherapy as might be indicated for a younger person. If you have other medical conditions such as heart trouble or diabetes, these can rule out certain chemotherapy treatments that might be recommended for people without those medical conditions.

When recommending a treatment, medical oncologists and other doctors look at something called the "risk-to-benefit ratio." In a nutshell, this means that doctors must mentally weigh all the possible health risks of a particular treatment against all its anticipated health benefits. Factors that come into play include how advanced and how rapidly growing your cancer is believed to be, and the statistical effectiveness of various courses of treatment and chemotherapy drugs. The possibility of achieving a remission, the effect of treatment on quality of life, the extension of life span, the mitigation of pain, and the potential damage of side effects are some of the variables that are weighed when deciding to recommend a particular course of treatment. Quality of life is an important consideration.

When the cure rate is low and survival is expected to be short, quality of life issues take on even more importance. Here are some questions to ask:

- When quality of life is considered, will chemotherapy treatments allow me to carry on everyday activities?
- Will they allow me to interact with my family?
- Will chemotherapy improve my ability to function?
- Will it alleviate pain, improve emotional conditions, allow for nutritional improvements, or provide relief from infection or bleeding?

If palliation of symptoms is the goal of your chemotherapy, and remission is not possible, this should be clearly explained to you.

Considering all these factors in addition to your physical condition might lead an oncologist to recommend treating high-risk breast cancer with an aggressive combination chemotherapy containing Adriamycin, which has a number of potential side effects, or a milder "CMF" therapy containing Cytoxan, methotrexate, and fluorouracil, which might be suitable for an older, frailer patient. As another example, a patient in the advanced stages of some cancers would also have to be in good physical condition before an oncologist would even consider recommending an expensive, experimental procedure such as an autologous bone marrow transplant, which makes very high-dose chemotherapy possible and offers a chance of achieving remission for some cancers that normally cannot be cured.

After explaining the risks and benefits of each treatment option, your oncologist will probably recommend a *treatment plan,* also called a treatment regimen, program, or protocol. Your treatment plan includes recommendations about which chemotherapy drugs to use, specific dosages, and the timing and sequence in which the anticancer drugs should be administered.

Understanding Your Options

The risks and benefits of each treatment option should be lucidly presented and carefully explained to you. You should consider yourself and your family an integral part of this process and this decision, because you all will live with the results of your decision.

Early on in this process, you might want to find out something about your medical oncologist's medical treatment philosophy. Does your doctor believe in aggressively battling cancer right to the end with chemotherapy treatments, or does he or she believe in stopping treatments fairly early if chemotherapy isn't producing the desired results? Which type of doctor would you prefer? Make sure you have a meeting of the minds on this issue, and that you clearly state your own preferences about such things as your wish to prolong or not to prolong your own life with "heroic" or extraordinary measures such as maintaining you on life-support systems. Whether you think you'll need it or not, you might want to draw up a legal document called a living will, clearly stating your wishes in this regard *before* you begin treatment.

Before you make this decision, you may want to consult the PDQ database by calling the toll-free number for the National Cancer Institute listed in the Other Resources appendix of this book. Tell the operator the type of cancer you have, and he or she will send you a free state-of-the-art cancer treatment summary for patients. This basic information includes a description of your cancer, explanations about how the cancer is staged, and brief explanations of options for treating each stage of cancer. From PDQ you may also request information about clinical trials to present to your doctor. At the present time, PDQ is set up to allow only medical doctors access to certain specific medical data on clinical trials, but you can help the process along by requesting the clinical trial data that's available to a person with your type and stage of cancer. Present a copy of this information to your doctor. Your doctor can look over the data and see if any ongoing clinical trials might be of potential interest or benefit to you.

Second Opinions

Some insurance companies require that patients secure a second opinion before treatment for cancer. Wendy Harpham, M.D., a doctor who underwent intensive chemotherapy and then wrote a book based on her own experiences, advises patients to seek a second opinion even if their treatment plan is fairly standard.

Dr. Harpham strongly advises people to seek a second opinion in the following situations:

- When multiple treatment options are available to you
- When significant risk is involved in your treatment
- When the treatment affects your existing lifestyle
- When you feel pushed into making a decision
- When you don't feel confident in the doctor or his or her recommended treatment

While doctors frequently agree with each other's recommendations, this is not always the case.

"My friends who worked at the Salk Clinic yelled and screamed at me. They *insisted* that I get a second opinion, and now I'm really glad that I listened to them," said one young mother, now free of colon cancer for more than two years. Taking the advice of her friends who worked at a cancer research laboratory, the patient sought a second opinion at a comprehensive cancer care hospital. After receiving a second opinion, she elected to receive a promising experimental treatment involving surgery, chemotherapy, and radiation for colon cancer rather than the standard surgical treatment recommended by her first doctor— which would have left her with a colostomy at the age of thirty-six.

Ask Questions

Some oncologists have been assessing the risks and benefits of particular treatments for such a long time that the process is something they no longer think completely through on a conscious level. They also may not explain how they arrived at a recommendation very clearly or very well. If necessary, it's your job to insist that the risks and benefits of all possible medical options be carefully explained to you in a way you can understand.

Since there is no national data bank containing information on all the people ever treated for cancer, clinical trial results are often used to estimate survival rates. These results can be expressed in different ways, so try to make sure that the same methods of calculating survival rates are used when different medical alternatives are compared. Some important factors to be examined when discussing clinical trial results include the stage of a particular cancer that patients had when they entered the study, the length of time results were measured after the study concluded, and if very many patients dropped out of the study before the follow-up results were measured and calculated. Unless you have a medical or scientific background, this array of facts will probably get very confusing. Most people simply rely on their medical oncologist to evaluate these results, but you do have the option to further research the facts and evaluate them yourself.

All the factors that your oncologist weighs are of potential interest to you. The results of tests done on you and their role in your diagnosis should be explained to you in as much detail as you care to hear. You have a right to understand *every one* of the treatment options your oncologist presents, and to hear the risks and benefits of each treatment to you. You also have the right to *not* ask any questions, if you are one of those people who is comfortable letting the doctor handle the medical nuances of your treatment.

Treatment Outcomes

As your doctor may or may not explain, chemotherapy is given only to accomplish one or more of the following five treatment outcomes:

Chemotherapy can cure cancer. By the term "cure," doctors normally mean that the patient will survive at least five years after being diagnosed with cancer. Most oncologists don't like the term cure, and prefer the term "in remission," which doesn't imply an ironclad promise that cancer won't recur. After cancer has been in remission for at least five years, survival rates for people who have had cancer usually approach normal rates for their sex and age groups.

Chemotherapy can stop cancer from spreading, or slow down its growth. Even when anticancer drugs don't completely kill all the cancerous cells in a particular tumor, chemotherapy can drastically slow down their growth and allow patients to live longer lives.

Chemotherapy can relieve symptoms caused by cancer. In some cases, symptoms such as pain from cancer can be relieved or palliated by chemotherapy treatments. For instance, chemotherapy in the form of estrogen tablets often relieves the bone pain caused by prostate cancer. A version of the CMF combination chemotherapy is sometimes used for palliation of advanced breast cancer.

Chemotherapy can shrink a tumor. Chemotherapy is sometimes used before surgery or radiation treatment to shrink the tumor so that it may be more easily and completely removed.

Chemotherapy can prevent cancer from recurring. After surgery or radiation, chemotherapy is sometimes used to "clean up" the small clumps of cancerous cells that may have spread to other parts of the body. This is also known as *adjuvant chemotherapy*.

Adjuvant therapy helps kill the small, nearly invisible colonies of cancer cells that may have spread to other sites even before they are large enough to detect. When there is a risk of a recurrent cancer, adjuvant chemotherapy can be one of the most successful forms of chemotherapy, and most effective if begun as soon as possible after surgery or radiation treatments.

Understand from the beginning which of these treatment outcomes is the ultimate goal of your chemotherapy. The goal of driving the cancer into remission is different from the goal of giving chemotherapy to palliate or relieve symptoms such as pain. Ask about the *prognosis* or expected result of your treatment. Unfortunately, patients sometimes don't hear medical treatment explanations clearly, and they can make assumptions that simply are not true. This may lead to disappointment and a feeling of betrayal. You and your family must have a realistic understanding of what your treatment actually seeks to achieve. Strive for clear communication between you as a patient and your medical team.

Questions to Ask

When your oncologist recommends a chemotherapy treatment, here are some things to be sure you understand, or ask about:

- How do you know for sure that I have cancer, and how did you determine which stage it is in?
- What are all the options for treatment available for treating this particular type of cancer, including investigational and conventional treatments?
- What are the cure rates for each treatment option?
- What are the short-term risks of each option?
- What are the long-term risks of each option?
- What side effects may be expected with each option?
- What is the risk of dying during treatment—for each option?
- How might each treatment affect my life, work, special interests, and so on?
- How long will each course of treatment last?
- Where should I go to receive each treatment, and who will administer it?
- What are the costs to me of each course of treatment?
- Will any of these treatments limit future treatment strategies?
- What is the risk of a second cancer occurring?
- What are the risks of additional medical problems from each course of treatment?
- How much time may I take to weigh or research these alternatives, without harming my chances for recovery?

You may want to tape record the answers to these questions, or bring someone along with you and have that person help you listen or take notes. You may want to think about the choices that you have for a while, until you feel most comfortable with one of them.

Response Rate

Since doctors can't predict how you will respond to a particular course of chemotherapy with complete accuracy, they will express your chances in terms of something called the *response rate*. The *response rate* is the percentage of people with your type of cancer who have had a favorable response to a particular course of treatment in the past.

If treatment option A has a 60 percent response rate, that doesn't mean that every tumor treated will shrink exactly 60 percent. It means that 60 percent of the people who have received that particular treatment in the past have been cured, or at least their cancer has gone into remission so that their life was extended at least five years. On the other side of that statistic, the remaining 40 percent had a negative response. People within this group may have experienced an incomplete remission, where the cancer did not continue to grow, or shrank but did not disappear.

Here are the four possible responses to chemotherapy treatment:

Complete remission. The cancer disappears without a visible trace, a complete remission. This is the response that everyone hopes for in every chemotherapy, including the patient and the doctor. Complete remission can happen before the end of chemotherapy treatment, but even if the cancer disappears, the chemotherapy is almost always continued through its course to prevent the relapses that may occur if treatment is stopped too soon.

Partial remission. The cancer shrinks but doesn't disappear. Chemotherapy may be continued, or another anticancer drug or drug combination may be tried. If the cancer stops shrinking, radiation or surgery is sometimes an option to remove the remaining cancer.

Stabilization. The tumor stabilizes, neither shrinking or growing. This period of stabilization may be brief, or it may last for many years.

Progression. The cancer continues to grow despite chemotherapy treatments. This response is the most difficult. After the chemotherapy treatments have had a fair chance to work, and if the cancer continues to grow, the doctor will want to explore a different treatment program.

Response Rate Statistics

Note that response rate statistics are only statistics. These statistics are calculated on the assumption that you have what is called a "functional status" of 70 percent or better.

The Karnofsky Performance Status scale is a way doctors have to measure your ability to function in the world, or your physical ability to live a normal life. If you function just fine in your life and work—for instance, if you are able to work and move around normally—then you have a functional status of 100 percent. If you are bedridden or nonfunctional half of the time, then you have a functional status of 50 percent, and so on. A Karnofsky Performance Status rating of zero would mean that you could not function at all.

According to Paul H. Coluzzi, M.D., regional medical director of Vitas Healthcare Corporation, the use of normal response rate statistics for patients who have a functional status of below 70 percent is clearly wrong. Bedridden patients with a low functional status will not have the same response rate to a particular treatment as people who are functioning normally, because bedridden patients are weaker than patients who are not bedridden. For patients with a low functional status, such as patients in rest homes, Dr. Coluzzi says response rate statistics must be examined with a skeptical eye because they may overstate the possible response.

Whether your cancer is growing quickly or slowly may factor into how much time you can allow yourself to make a decision about medical treatment. With a fast-growing cancer, you may have to act quickly. Since there are no guaranteed cures with chemotherapy, understand that you may never feel 100 percent comfortable with the option you choose. But also understand that any treatment option you choose may very well rid your body of cancer.

Medical Tests

Chemotherapy has risks and benefits, and so do medical tests. Certainly, you will be tested very frequently—first to establish a baseline for further tests, then to determine the stage of your cancer, and finally to monitor the response of your body to the chemotherapy treatments. Expect to be tested more times than you would like. You should understand the value of the medical tests you are given.

Medical tests are inconvenient for the patient, occasionally painful, and they do cost money. As a general rule, invasive tests that occur inside your skin are a bit more risky than noninvasive tests that have almost no risk if properly done. Unfortunately, some tests may have to be redone, which is an annoying development—for instance, if your x-rays weren't perfectly clear the first time around. Somewhere in the middle of your chemotherapy treatment, you may just feel as if you have had all the medical tests you wish to have for the rest of your life.

Your oncologist should be balancing the toll these tests take on your body and spirit against the anticipated benefit of the information each test will ultimately provide. If you don't understand the value of a particular test, ask to have it explained to you. Your doctor should be able to explain how any test is useful. You also have a right to know your test results, if you wish. You may ask if the results of a particular test will make any difference or not to your treatment, or whether each test is medically necessary. If it's not necessary, why take it? You should also understand that if you decline to take tests that your oncologist feels are necessary, you might be depriving your health-care team of information which could affect your recovery.

Your Options

The treatment plan you ultimately approve will include not only one or more chemotherapy drugs, but also a schedule for chemotherapy treatment.

Sometimes the options you are presented may seem like a choice between bad and worse. With the exception of most skin cancers and *in situ* ovarian cancer, you won't be offered the possibility of an almost certain cure. Certainly, the decision to select a particular treatment option can vary from individual to individual. There may even be differences of opinion within the family, which will add to the anguish and confusion.

Many patients want to "go for broke," and go for their best chance for a cure by trying the harshest, most aggressive possible course of chemotherapy presented—regardless of the possible risks. Some people might prefer a shorter life and a peaceful death at home to the costs and complications of a particular course of treatment that offers only a short extension of life, with many possible side effects. Some people will want to participate in a clinical trial. Others would never consider leaving their hometown for treatment of any disease. The variables of every decision are unique.

Response rate statistics are important because they give you some idea of how effective a particular course of treatment might be. Side effects vary considerably from person to person, but it helps if you have a generally positive attitude and don't release your will to live. Don't ever give up hope. If you take very good care of yourself during treatment, your chances of survival may be better than what the latest response rate statistics (already several years old) might indicate.

Informed Consent

Before you begin chemotherapy treatments, you will be asked to sign an informed consent form. This document describes the recommended treatment, its expected benefits, and also all the possible side effects that can occur with the chemotherapy and from particular drugs. Carefully reading your informed consent form may just take your breath away, because your doctor is legally required to list every known complication that could possibly occur, including those that happen very rarely. The consent form you sign may be even more ominous if you participate in a clinical trial, where the guidelines of the U.S. Department of Health's policy regarding protection of human research subjects comes into play.

But if you want the chemotherapy, you must sign this form. Plan to receive and keep a copy of what you have signed. Understand that the informed consent form is designed for the legal protection of the doctor, and to fully inform the patient about the risks of medical treatment. Its purpose is not to put your mind at ease about a particular course of treatment. It is merely a legal document that states that you have been warned of all the possible risks your treatment might involve. It may put your mind at ease to ask your doctor or nurse which side effects listed on the informed consent form are likely to occur, as many side effects may be very rare. In the case of children with cancer, parents or legal guardians must sign the consent form. Again, ask what side effects are likely to occur. In the special case of children, Supreme Court decisions have held that courts may order a life-saving treatment for a child even if the parents wish the treatment withheld for religious or other reasons.

If you are an adult, of course you have the right to refuse chemotherapy. It is understood that without medical treatment, your cancer will take a fairly predictable course, which can be explained to you. Spontaneous remissions do occur once in a blue moon, but they are very rare. Only a few hundred have been documented. If you do not choose chemotherapy, ask your doctor about painkilling drugs and other methods of relieving the pain you may experience. Ask about antinausea drugs, since nausea can be a side effect of cancer. Understand that if you refuse chemotherapy, blood transfusions may be needed at some point, and you may benefit from radiation therapy of the affected areas to help reduce pain and other symptoms of cancer. Please discuss your decision not to accept chemotherapy with your physician, since it is possible he or she may be able to help make the remainder of your life easier and more pleasant. As chapter 19 explains, unorthodox medical treatments like laetrile or megavitamin therapy may be painless, and they may sound great, but they aren't a viable substitute for chemotherapy.

Nagging Doubts

Even after you've chosen a method of treatment that includes chemotherapy, you may continue to have doubts as to whether you're "doing the right thing." Chemotherapy can be an unpleasant experience with attendant side effects. Your oncologist can't give you an ironclad guarantee that the treatment plan you choose to follow will work, even though you have a reasonable hope that success or improvement will occur.

Take comfort in knowing that fear or anxiety is a normal emotional reaction. Adding to your apprehension about the course of treatment you have chosen, you may hear stories over the back fence, or in the doctor's office waiting room. In the waiting room, you may meet people with the same kind of cancer you have being treated differently than you. These stories may frighten you, and make you inclined to question your doctor's judgment. Since it's your only body that's at risk here, you can't expect to purchase medical treatment as comfortably as you would buy a new car, a new computer, or a new hat.

When in doubt, ask more questions.

Children with Cancer

Childhood cancer is fortunately quite rare, comprising less than 1 percent of the diagnosed cancer cases in North America each year. Leukemias and lymphomas are the most common forms of childhood cancer, but other cancers such as neuroblastoma, Wilms' tumor, bone, and brain cancers occur with some frequency in young children. Most of the time, the families of the approximately ten thousand American children diagnosed each year with childhood cancer become intimately involved with the cancer therapy—so much so that childhood cancer is often called "a family disease." Parents must understand and approve the medical treatment for the child, transport the child to and from treatment, often care for the child at home, and bear the financial and emotional burdens in a way that is different from adults who may often help themselves.

Good cancer treatment for children frequently involves the coordination of many medical specialists such as pediatric medical oncologists, pediatric surgeons, and hematologists. Since childhood cancer is fairly rare, by far the best cure rates are achieved at pediatric hospitals where these types of cancers are seen and treated on a day-to-day basis. Pediatric hospitals are normally friendly, upbeat places, accustomed to working with and caring for children, and well able to provide for the special needs of children, such as the need to play. Near many pediatric hospitals are Ronald McDonald Houses or other houses or apartments where families can stay for a low cost, and interact with and support other families who have family members in the hospital.

Fortunately, as with many cancers, remission rates for many types of childhood cancer have improved quite dramatically in the past few years. For instance, the five-year survival rate for acute lymphocytic leukemia has increased from just 4 percent in the early 1960s to 70 percent in the 1980s. The cure rate for osteosarcoma increased from 20 percent to 50 percent during the same period of time.

Is Chemotherapy Working?

Most of the time chemotherapy drugs begin to show some effect within four to ten weeks. Some chemotherapy treatments used for cancers such as breast cancer, however, may require several months' time before results are noticeable. Each individual's response time to treatment may also vary. With adjuvant therapy used after surgery or radiation against tumors too small to detect, you may not ever know for sure that the treatment worked, although cancer never reappears.

Nobody expects you to like any of the side effects of cancer treatment, or to enjoy the social trauma that you and your family may well undergo. Although you can overdo it, it's healthy to complain a little bit when you are ill. Receiving chemotherapy treatment for cancer may upset your emotional or social life, but chapter 16 surveys some of the stress-relieving techniques you can use to help yourself get through to the other side of wellness.

Remember that the enemy is cancer. Chemotherapy may shock your system or rock your metabolism, but it is your ally in what may be one of the major battles of your entire life. Give yourself a chance to defeat cancer by seeing your treatment through, and work to get well. The next chapter discusses where chemotherapy is administered, and explains the risks and the benefits of participating in clinical trials.

6

WHERE YOU MIGHT RECEIVE CHEMOTHERAPY

AT A BIG CANCER TREATMENT CENTER, OR CLOSER TO HOME?

DEPENDING ON SEVERAL FACTORS, INCLUDING THE TYPE OF CHEMOTHERAPY you receive, you may receive chemotherapy at a large comprehensive cancer center, which offers specialized treatment, or at a smaller facility, which may be closer to your home. Clinical trials are sometimes an option. This chapter explains clinical trials and explains how to locate trials, which might be appropriate.

Your choice of where you receive chemotherapy treatments is often bound up with your selection of a medical oncologist who practices in a particular location. The two basic choices as to where to receive chemotherapy treatments are:

1. From a medical oncologist in private practice in your hometown, who may give you chemotherapy in his or her office, or at another location because of an affiliation with a particular hospital or managed care facility

2. From medical oncologists practicing in a big urban cancer center where new research is done, where many prominent physicians practice, and where treatment is state-of-the-art because all the doctors there treat nothing but cancer

Whatever you decide, remember that you can get good treatment in either situation. You can expect to get good cancer care from any board-certified oncologist, whose credentials may be verified by calling your local medical association, or the National Cancer Institute.

Give a little thought to which treatment environment you might prefer, and where you would feel most comfortable, because your attitude is important to your recovery. Since you'll be spending some time there while you're not feeling very well, plan to visit the facility beforehand. If the environment feels friendly, that's a good sign. A pleasant and friendly staff is important, and so is relatively prompt service without an inordinate amount of waiting time. If you'll be staying in a hospital, make sure the rooms are clean and well kept. Is it possible for your spouse or family members to stay in the room, or to find lodging nearby? If it's a long stay, even little things such as convenient parking may make a difference, as will your own need for things like flexible visiting hours, or rules allowing your personal mementos or property in the room. If your child is being treated for cancer, check for a facility like a Ronald McDonald House near the pediatric hospital. Most hospitals have lists of available housing near the hospital, which they provide upon request.

Scattered around the country, under the umbrella of the U.S. Department of Health's National Cancer Institute (NCI) cancer centers program, are several state-of-the-art comprehensive cancer centers which include such well-known names as Memorial Sloan-Kettering Cancer Center in New York, the Johns Hopkins Oncology Center in Baltimore, Maryland, the Mayo Comprehensive Cancer Center in Rochester, Minnesota, the University of Texas M. D. Anderson Center in Houston, Texas, or the Fred Hutchinson Cancer Research Center in Seattle, Washington.

The nearly thirty comprehensive cancer centers that have received NCI designation in the United States have developed outstanding reputations for good reason, the foremost of which is that their doctors have cured a lot of people of cancer. Comprehensive cancer centers meet important criteria such as the ability to transfer research findings into clinical practice. They all employ a multidisciplinary approach in the treatment of cancer that involves both medical treatment and what are called support services. Another eighteen NCI-approved clinical cancer centers such as the City of Hope National Medical Center in Duarte, California, also conduct research and treat patients.

Most oncologists who practice at cancer centers have collectively supervised or participated in a lot of important research that has helped advance the science of medicine. Major cancer centers typically have billing offices that handle much of the financial paperwork for you. A complete list of cancer centers may be acquired by calling the National Cancer Institute, whose toll-free telephone number is listed in the Other Resources appendix of this book.

Pros and Cons

Here are some advantages of being treated at a large cancer center:

- *Expertise.* The oncologists who practice at these centers have amassed a great deal of experience, even with very rare cancers.
- *Latest methods.* Evaluation and treatment methods may be presumed to be modern and up-to-date for all types of cancer, including those that are uncommon or very advanced. You will also have access to specialists in fields such as blood banking to help manage any complications caused by chemotherapy.
- *New treatments.* Investigational programs and clinical trials are offered that may be a bit more effective than standard treatments.

Disadvantages include:

- *Impersonality.* You might not have one doctor caring for you, but a number of physicians who follow a similar protocol or method of treating you. This may include receiving treatment from oncology fellows, young cancer doctors in training without a lot of actual experience, who are nonetheless supervised by an experienced staff oncologist.

- *Loneliness.* You may not see much of your friends and family during treatment, if it is inconvenient to visit you in a distant location.
- *Expense.* The cost of traveling and being away from home for periods of time should be added to the emotional "expense" of moving back and forth for a period of time. If a friend or spouse accompanies you, they will also have travel and lodging expenses, which probably won't be covered by insurance.
- *Referral.* Another doctor's referral is needed.

For rare cancers where treatment involves a number of specialists who coordinate their efforts on a treatment plan, a large cancer center is probably the best bet because most doctors may only see such cancers once or twice in their careers.

This is true in the case of children with cancer, where multimodality treatments including chemotherapy are common, and where a recognized pediatric hospital staffed with pediatric oncologists is almost always advised because cure rates are much higher. In the United States and Canada, the Children's Cancer Study Group and the Pediatric Oncology Group are two cooperative groups that treat most cases of pediatric cancer in "centers of excellence," which are approved pediatric cancer specialty units. All children treated in a center of excellence, and their parents, are asked to participate in clinical trials.

When considering where to receive treatment, the time involved in particular chemotherapy treatments is another factor to consider, as is the length of time it will take to complete the treatments. You may want to check your health insurance policy—travel and lodging expenses by family members are typically not covered, nor is treatment in most clinical trials.

At some point during some chemotherapy treatments, you may be able to come home and receive chemotherapy. Many insurance companies encourage this, since it's less expensive than staying in a hospital. If possible, receiving chemotherapy at home will involve lining up the necessary medical equipment, and probably some amount of home nursing care. You may need to arrange for visiting oncology nurses to come to your home. Your care will involve the cooperation of your family, who can take home care courses taught in some hospitals. It may be possible to coordinate all these factors, or it may not.

At any rate, your local doctor may advise you as to whether a trip to a big cancer center is worthwhile. Some interesting clinical trials may be underway in some cancer centers for promising new treatments for your type and stage of cancer. If you have an interest, ask your doctor about clinical trials and investigate them carefully before you begin chemotherapy.

Clinical Trials

Over the past few decades, hundreds of thousands of drugs have been screened for their effectiveness as anticancer agents in clinical trials. The selection process is rigorous and thorough and most drugs are eliminated. Although nearly ten thousand different chemicals are in tests each year, new anticancer agents are not approved unless their benefits in fighting cancer clearly and definitively outweigh their risks.

The testing process involves several levels of tests. First, the drugs are tested in test tubes containing cancer cells, formally known as antineoplastic drug screens. If the drug reduces the number of cancer cells in test tubes, it may be tested for toxicity on mice with tumors. These animal tests give research scientists some idea of possible side effects as well as an idea of effective dosage levels for human beings. Sometimes, primates such as monkeys are used for testing the effects of drugs before they are cleared for human testing.

After tumor-reducing benefits are shown to exist in animal tests, a drug is cleared to go into human subject trials. The drug's official sponsor, usually the National Cancer Institute, files an application to test the drug with the U.S. Food and Drug Administration (FDA). The FDA application includes the results of tests already completed. Ultimately, the FDA must approve anticancer drugs for medical use after they have gone through three levels of clinical trials on human subjects and passed them all with acceptable results.

Phase I trials test anticancer drugs used on humans for the first time. Phase I trials are *toxicity* studies that seek to determine the maximum dose a human can withstand before unacceptable side effects occur. Some drugs are weeded out after this stage of testing, which is also the phase at which the most unacceptable side effects in humans such as severe liver or kidney damage may well occur. Frequently, patients in Phase I and Phase II trials are those with advanced cancers such as lung, pancreas, and kidney cancer on whom other drugs did not work.

Phase II trials involve drugs that have passed through Phase I trials and still show promise. Phase II trials are *efficacy* trials seeking to find the drug's effectiveness against several types of cancer.

Finally, Phase III trials seek to determine if the new drugs that passed through the first two levels of trials are more effective than standard treatments. Normally, Phase III trials have a control group of cancer patients receiving the standard treatment, and compare those results against a group receiving the new treatment, although sometimes research scientists may use a "historical" comparison in which they compare the results of treatment with the new drug against historical records of standard treatment regimens. Only drugs that scientists believe may prove *better* than standard treatments are tested in Phase III trials.

If a new drug appears better than the standard treatment and has passed all its tests, then a new drug application is filed with the FDA, which must approve the drug before it can be marketed. This process takes several years, long after the anticancer drug has passed Phase I, Phase II, and Phase III trials.

When to Consider a Clinical Trial

If no other effective treatment exists for your cancer, you may want to consider participating in a clinical trial. A benefit of participating in a clinical trial is that it often provides the comfort of knowing you may be helping future cancer patients by your participation. Treatment is usually free, but most patients agree that cost alone is *not* sufficient reason to participate in any clinical trial. Also, some oncologists who are experts in certain types of cancer will not treat patients with new drugs outside the framework of a clinical trial. It is possible that you will randomly be placed in the control group in your clinical trial, and receive a standard protocol of chemotherapy rather than the experimental drug treatment.

The downside of clinical trials is that you may receive little benefit from the treatment. In fact, you may risk suffering more side effects than with a standard regimen. Even though your chemotherapy bills are typically paid for because you are participating in an experiment, you or your family may have travel expenses and other expenses getting to and from the hospital that will not be reimbursed. Additional tests may also be necessary to evaluate the effectiveness of the experimental drug after treatment, so you should fully understand the scope of what's expected of you.

It is almost always best to begin your treatment for cancer with the standard recommended chemotherapy, because it probably has the greatest chance of being successful. Certainly, you would want to think long and hard before entering a Phase I or even a Phase II trial, even if your cancer is not responding to standard chemotherapy. Any decision such as this should be made after consultation with your doctor. You will need to understand what costs you may be responsible for, including costs for treatments needed to correct side effects of experimental therapy. And don't forget to check with your insurance company, since many health insurance companies refuse to pay for therapies using drugs or therapies that they consider experimental.

Local Care

If you are the type of person who likes to stay at home and be close to your family, you might prefer that a good local oncologist treat you. Your local oncologist can sometimes discuss your case over the telephone with doctors at major cancer centers, which can be of some benefit to you. Note that the PDQ database is available to any oncologist—make sure your doctor knows about it. If your chemotherapy treatment is not complex, or is one with which your local oncologist has had experience and success, you might decide to stay close to home and save yourself and perhaps your family members the economic and emotional stress of traveling back and forth to a larger facility.

Oncologists in cancer centers carefully follow specific protocols, or standardized sequences of treatment for the various types of cancer. Big cancer centers follow treatment protocols *because* they do research—having standard protocols helps them in evaluating and measuring research results, and to compare results from standard and experimental treatment methods.

Oncologists in private practice, on the other hand, have a bit more freedom. They can customize their treatment to the individual patient to a greater extent, and their level of personal attention and interaction with you will probably be higher than at a large facility. A single physician may be able to follow your personal progress a bit more closely than a team of doctors at a cancer center who collaborate on your care.

The decision as to where you wish to receive chemotherapy is important. But whether you receive chemotherapy in a comprehensive cancer center or from a private medical oncologist, you won't just be treated by any one person. You'll be interacting with a great number of men and women who will comprise your medical treatment team.

7

YOUR MEDICAL TREATMENT TEAM

Some Specialists You Might Meet during Your Treatment

Receiving chemotherapy brings you into contact with a number of medical specialists and technicians who perform specific tasks or duties. This is your medical treatment team. You can think of them as a symphony orchestra or a dance band if you like, but realize that each individual has a slightly different part to play in the highly coordinated effort that is your treatment.

Sometimes, especially if you are being treated by several specialists in a large cancer center, it may be difficult to keep the medical specialists straight, and to understand who to ask about what. In addition to all the medical specialists, you may meet other professionals such as psychologists or social workers who play a role in your care.

Interaction with so many people can be quite bewildering. In the middle of all the fast-moving white, green, and blue jackets, you may feel like standing up and shouting, "Who's in charge here?"

Theoretically, the cancer treatment team is headed by *the patient*. After all, nobody knows how you feel better than you. You're the world expert on your medical history, what you can tolerate and not tolerate, where you hurt, and so forth. You have the option of choosing your treatment or even refusing to be treated for cancer at all. You are the one who may solicit a second or even a third medical opinion. You're the orchestra conductor. Although you may not feel like it, you're actually the captain of the great white ship that holds your entire treatment team.

Form a Partnership

Doctors are your team's medical and scientific experts, and their expertise should be acknowledged. For their years of study and experience, respect their medical judgment. Your case is most important, particularly to you. Realize, though, that doctors deal with a tremendous volume of people, and they are taught in medical school to cope with the demands of their profession by keeping a professional distance. They do this to protect themselves, but this distance can be felt and it makes some doctors very hard to warm up to. Although there is more than a little arrogance and brusqueness in the world of specialized medicine, the M.D. after a person's name does not stand for "Medical Deity." Doctors are only people, after all, and they don't walk on water. You don't have to worship them. You don't even have to like them very much. The bottom line is that you should respect your doctor's medical judgment and have some confidence that he or she has the skill to help you heal.

"Form a partnership with your physician or other healing professional, rather than an employer/employee relationship with you as the employee," advises Harold Benjamin, author of *From Victim to Victor*. Although Benjamin believes in the healing power of support groups such as the Wellness Community, he stresses the importance of following your doctor's advice. Benjamin advises cancer patients, "Know that you are not helpless and that you are the most important member of the team fighting for recovery."

Note, too, that you often become the bridge between the medical team and your family members and friends who want to know what is happening to you. You may have to answer some medical questions, or to explain cancer to a child. You also have the responsibility to inform other health professionals, such as your dentist, that you are undergoing chemotherapy treatments. Most importantly, you will receive the chemotherapy and you will deal with its intimate effects on your own body.

Yes, you are theoretically the head of this partnership or team. But the idea that you will receive chemotherapy treatments may still make you fear that you have lost all control over your life. You may feel like a deer in the forest, hearing the first clap of thunder that signals a powerful thunderstorm. Understanding who you will meet and what procedures you may experience will help you feel more in control of the process.

Learning about your treatment requires that you ask questions of your medical team, and that you listen carefully to the answers. Medical specialists are busy people. Specialists are trained to look not at the person, but at the disease. Their relationships with patients are typically not as long as the relationship between a patient and a family doctor, which might last many decades. To get the full attention of a busy specialist, you may have to be like the enterprising patient who posted a little sign over her hospital bed that read, "Don't forget—I am a human being."

Communicate

To receive complete information, you'll have to assert yourself. Hone your ability to ask questions. Don't be afraid to ask questions of your oncologist, your cancer nurse, or anyone else you encounter. Keep asking questions until you feel you understand your treatment, understand what side effects to anticipate, and feel convinced you know some ways to mitigate their effects. You'll have to assert yourself, often, because medical professionals wait for cues from patients that they are ready to discuss their treatment program openly. Doctors know that they have some patients who don't wish to know *any* of the details of their treatment. Or sometimes people need a lot of time to work things through. Therefore, if you want immediate answers, be prepared to ask questions and demand answers from your medical team.

Most specialists try to follow the latest research in their field, and keep up on new treatments and new developments. If you want to make sure your oncologist has all the latest information on treatments for your particular type of cancer, ask that he or she consult the Physicians' Data Query (PDQ) maintained by the National Cancer Institute, whose toll-free telephone number is listed in the Other Resources appendix of this book. A computerized query of the PDQ database will quickly yield a trove of information on the latest treatment methods, drugs, or promising treatments being evaluated in clinical trials. Some of this information might be useful in developing the most effective treatment plan for your cancer. If you request it, your oncologist will share the less technical portion of the PDQ report with you. You can also request a free state-of-the-art treatment summary for your type of cancer from PDQ and present it to your doctor.

Trust

Because you are embarking on a serious course of action, you must ultimately trust your oncologist's medical judgment about chemotherapy. If you have any doubts, even after you have begun chemotherapy, seek a second medical doctor's opinion. You might even want to ask your doctor for a referral to another physician. Be upfront if you wish a second opinion—enlist your doctor's help, don't sneak around behind his or her back. A little anxiety is normal at this point, and you'll have to accept that. The bottom line is: Find a physician whose medical judgment you trust.

Doctors don't read minds, so do give your doctor a chance to understand your concerns and to respond to your questions. At the very least, you should feel that you can openly communicate with your doctor, because you want a relationship built on mutual trust. You have the responsibility to put your concerns into words or to get someone to ask questions for you. If you experience a medical problem during treatment, ask your doctor or your nurse what you can do about it. Assert yourself, because it will help you. It is possible that you'll find one person on the medical treatment team that you trust most, and you may want to ask that person some of your more personal questions.

Medical Specialists

Since cancer is complex, being treated for cancer requires that you see a lot of doctors with various specialties.

Your primary care physician has probably referred you to at least one oncologist who specializes in the treatment of cancer. Within this field are many subspecialties. *Medical oncologists,* who are sometimes called *chemotherapists,* are the physicians who actually recommend a course of chemotherapy, and choose the anticancer drugs and treatment schedule. Medical oncologists have years of advanced training in both internal medicine and in the judicious use of anticancer drugs. Among doctors, medical oncologists are the acknowledged experts on the arsenal of drugs used to control cancer, and on drugs that can mitigate particular side effects.

If you are receiving multimodality treatment that involves several specialists, your medical oncologist will likely be the person who coordinates the activities of the other specialists, primarily because he or she will be seeing you for a much more extended period of time. In a managed care or health maintenance organization (HMO) setting, the medical care team is structured differently. In an HMO, the primary care physician is usually the hub of the treatment wheel for all medical treatments including treatment for cancer.

Medical oncologists treat most types of cancer most of the time. Exceptions are prostate cancer where a *urologist* more typically coordinates the medical activities of specialists, and gynecological cancer where a *gynecological oncologist* usually oversees both chemotherapy and surgery. From time to time, chemotherapy is given by surgical oncologists, or blood disease specialists called *hematologists.*

With multimodality treatments, *radiation oncologists* administer radiation therapy. *Surgical oncologists* perform cancer surgery. Surgeons may be called in early on to perform tasks such as obtaining the tissue necessary for a biopsy, which is the only real way to confirm a diagnosis for almost all cancers. Surgeons also surgically remove tumors, sometimes freezing the tumor, or using high-tech tools such as microwaves or lasers. *Pathologists* analyze the structural and functional changes caused by disease to your body, like detectives examining slides of tissue samples to calculate the state of your disease.

Pediatric oncologists specialize in the treatment of children with cancer.

In chemotherapy treatment, you may find that an important and high-profile member of the medical team is the *oncology nurse* or cancer nurse. The oncology nurse administers the actual chemotherapy treatments and works closely with the entire medical team in either a hospital, a private medical office setting, or in the home where people sometimes receive chemotherapy.

Other medical specialists you may encounter include *pharmacists* who fill prescriptions for drugs or medications, and *medical technicians* or *lab technicians* who actually administer some tests and analyze their results.

After treatment, *rehabilitation therapists* may help patients with particular problems move back toward a normal life. For instance, people treated for cancer of the larynx may need to relearn how to talk. *Physical therapists* help patients exercise and strengthen muscles after they have been in bed or immobilized for long periods of time, since lack of exercise weakens muscles that are not regularly used. Physical therapists also work with patients who might need to learn how to use an artificial limb. *Plastic surgeons* are doctors who work with patients who require reconstructive surgery, such as the reconstruction of a breast after surgery for breast cancer.

Beyond the purely medical, *social workers,* often stationed at hospitals, can help patients and families cope with social, practical, and financial problems that come up during cancer treatment. *Nutritionists* recommend good nutritional strategies to help you get through chemotherapy by assuring that your body is as strong as possible before and during a particular course of chemotherapy. *Dieticians* plan meals that help cancer patients deal with the effects of chemotherapy.

Psychologists and *hospital chaplains* are counselors who may help you deal with emotional problems either in a hospital setting or as an outpatient.

THINGS TO DO BEFORE STARTING CHEMOTHERAPY

Here are a few things you might want to do before starting chemotherapy:

- Get a second medical opinion. Many health insurance policies require this, even for a course of treatment that is fairly standard.

- Begin to build up your physical strength and stamina as much as you can with moderate exercise and good nutrition. You may wish to consult a personal trainer, a nutritionist, or to request free booklets from the American Cancer Society or Cancer Information Service, which provide specific tips for managing cancer treatment.

- Provide your doctor with a list of the drugs you are currently taking, even those you consider harmless such as vitamin supplements, alcohol, and aspirin, because some of these can interfere with the workings of some chemotherapy drugs.

- Go to the dentist or periodontist and have your teeth cleaned and checked and cavities filled.

- Make sure your health insurance premiums are paid up to date, and that you have a copy of the most current benefits information and a supply of medical forms.

- Make a living will if you do not wish "heroic" medical treatment measures applied, and update your will to make sure your wishes are known. As much as possible, get your financial house in order.

- Educate yourself about which anticancer drugs might be used in your treatment, what some of the side effects might be, and some of the ways to plan for or mitigate the possible side effects. For instance, you can get fitted for a wig if your treatment has a possible side effect of hair loss—it's easier to match the color when the wig person can actually see the color and texture of your natural hair.

- Discuss the possible changes in your lifestyle with your family and friends. If you are going into the hospital for a period of time to receive chemotherapy, for instance, talk about such things as who will do the household chores, manage the finances, or take care of small children.

- Learn a bit more about what chemotherapy is and how chemotherapy treatments might affect your physical health, your social life, and your outlook on life. Learn everything you can do to make the process easier on you and your family.

Designated Person

If you have a big family or a lot of friends, it's a good idea to designate one person to interface with the medical team. This designated person doesn't have to be you. It is one thing for a doctor or a nurse to explain your situation to one relative, but it's quite another to expect your medical professionals to cover exactly the same material with a dozen more.

It is frequently a good idea to bring a spouse, an adult friend, or relative to your consultations or meetings with the doctor, to help you hear what the doctor is saying. But it's a poor idea to bring young children into the chemotherapist's office because it's not a safe environment for them. Children may bring in germs that can endanger other patients receiving chemotherapy whose immune systems are depressed.

Your medical team is of fundamental importance in your medical treatment. If you understand the roles of all the specialists you meet, it can make you more comfortable with chemotherapy. Now you are ready to examine the actual process of receiving chemotherapy treatments, which the next chapter covers.

8

RECEIVING CHEMOTHERAPY

How You May Receive Chemotherapy Treatments

ACTUALLY RECEIVING CHEMOTHERAPY INVOLVES SEVERAL CYCLES OF receiving chemotherapy drugs, alternating with periods where your body rests and recuperates. This chapter deals with how chemotherapy treatments are given, an aspect of treatment that frightens many people although perhaps it should not.

In the past ten years, more and more chemotherapy has been administered in an outpatient setting, that is, in a hospital without a formal hospital admission, or in a medical oncologist's office. Receiving chemotherapy treatments as an outpatient makes chemotherapy much like a normal visit to the doctor, where you wait in a waiting room, look at magazines, then proceed to smaller rooms where you may receive a blood test, consult with your doctor, and then receive chemotherapy treatment from an oncology nurse. Under the supervision of a doctor, chemotherapy treatments may sometimes be given in your home.

Chemotherapy treatments may take as little as fifteen minutes, or more than eight hours, depending on the drugs and the treatment program. These days, the average is about an hour and a half. Although some chemotherapy still must be administered in a hospital, some treatments are now so quick and simple that they can be administered during your lunch hour, after which you just get up and return to work.

Technological improvements include the small, portable ambient infusion pump. This small pump can deliver chemotherapy treatments for as long as a week. About the size of a pack of playing cards, it's already sophisticated enough to deliver as many as four separate anticancer drugs in a preset sequence. This technology allows patients to receive chemotherapy without being confined to a hospital.

Central venous catheters (thin, clear plastic tubes) are now installed in more than one-third of all patients receiving chemotherapy in some major cancer centers. The use of catheters helps prevent problems associated with collapsed veins, a particular problem in older patients.

Medically, new tools are available to mitigate chemotherapy's side effects. New colony-stimulating factors such as G-CSF, GM-CSF, and erythropoietin stimulate the growth of white or red blood cells, and lessen the side effects of fatigue and infection associated with some chemotherapy treatments.

Oncology Nurses

Oncology nurses, or cancer nurses, sit in the room with you when you are receiving chemotherapy to monitor your progress. You'll probably have a better chance to get to know the oncology nurse than the oncologist, because you'll spend more time in the nurse's company.

Good oncology nurses are sympathetic people who can be a resource for other specialists such as home care nurses. They know where to get things like hospital beds when they are needed. Cancer nurses are a direct line of communication to the doctor. They may report medical developments that come up in conversations when you are receiving chemotherapy, sometimes an important detail that you simply forgot to mention to the doctor.

Oncology nurses work with patients and their families to minimize problems related to medical treatment. Nurses are good sources for practical suggestions in coping with the physical side effects of chemotherapy. As a member of your medical treatment team, nurses may also refer you to social workers, dieticians, psychologists, or may provide information about support groups for either patients or family members.

In large comprehensive cancer centers, oncology nurses are trained to administer chemotherapy, to take blood for blood tests, and to communicate particular problems that their patients may be having to doctors. In smaller hospitals and private offices, oncology nurses may have additional duties, such as collecting urine specimens and mixing chemotherapy drugs, duties that would be performed by laboratory technicians and pharmacists in larger settings.

Oncology nurses typically wear a lot of protective clothing, such as rubber gloves, gowns, and sometimes face masks. Don't take this ominous, operating room look too personally. Oncology nurses wear protective clothing because of the multiple exposures to many types of drugs they encounter over the course of their work.

Some drugs used in chemotherapy are actually carcinogenic, their use regulated by the federal Occupational and Safety Health Administration (OSHA). Oncology nurses take sensible precautions with their own health because they are exposed to these drugs so frequently.

A note of caution: Remember that the nurse who gives you chemotherapy should be trained in cancer treatment, training that includes a study of both the drugs used and the treatment of side effects that may occur. In other words, he or she should be a trained oncology nurse. One patient recalls receiving chemotherapy from a "substitute" nurse who sought to save herself time by giving Adriamycin in a drip method rather than via a syringe. The patient's veins shut down, she was stuck in five places before it was over, and she couldn't straighten her arm for a month afterward. The moral to this story is: If the person giving you chemotherapy is not an oncology nurse, stand up and assert your right to be treated by a nurse who has been trained in the treatment of cancer.

Receiving Chemotherapy

Chemotherapy is administered in several ways, including orally—in pill, liquid, or other form. A lot of chemotherapy is given by injection, a technique called IV that is short for intravenous, or through the vein.

Chemotherapy given intravenously is most frequently given in the back of the hand or lower arm, rather than inside the forearm where blood samples are taken. Certainly, no person enjoys being swabbed with alcohol and then having their veins poked. It is a maddening experience to even *begin* chemotherapy if you are a person with small veins and the nurse has a problem finding a good vein. Sometimes there's a particular nurse in the office who is really good at finding your vein, and you might request to have that person always administer your chemotherapy even if it means changing your appointment time.

More and more, a *catheter* is placed under the skin to minimize the hassle of getting shots. A catheter can stay in for some time. It is hard to pull out, but it does need to be cleaned periodically with heparin, a drug that prevents blood clotting. A catheter can help you avoid the annoyance of having some nurse poke your skin every time you need a chemotherapy injection, a nutritional formula, a blood transfusion, or even painkilling drugs.

A more complicated version of the catheter called a venous access device (VAD) may be surgically inserted into the body—another way around the continual process of finding veins, drawing blood, and injecting medications during chemotherapy. Implanted infusion ports may be surgically placed under the skin, and they can greatly simplify chemotherapy treatment.

Common Fears

Even when you're in roaring good health, it's a common response to catch your breath when you see a cold, shining stainless steel needle. You may feel a twinge of apprehension when you step into a doctor's office and smell the medicinal odor of rubbing alcohol. If you feel frightened or apprehensive in these situations, know that you are not alone. Try to remember that the enemy is not the needle that brings the chemotherapy, but the cancer that all this medical paraphernalia is marshaled to treat. You may sit in a lot of cold rooms, and read a lot of boring magazines, but your medical treatment will have a beginning and an end. If all goes well, your chemotherapy treatments will someday be just a fading memory in your life.

If you're nervous, talk to other people such as nurses, friends, or family members about your treatment. Educate yourself—learn more about your chemotherapy and how to keep yourself in top physical shape while undergoing treatment. Participating in any way will help you feel more in control of your medical treatment. One way to participate is to try some of the stress reduction exercises in chapter 16, before, during, or after chemotherapy treatments.

One of the best ways to calm your apprehension about chemotherapy treatments is to take another person with you. This person, your "personal advocate," will help mitigate your anxiety, and it's always nice to have company. This is a particularly good idea for the first treatment when you don't know if any side effects will occur. If you're not feeling well, your personal advocate may be able to help deal with some of the red tape you encounter, such as medical and insurance forms and questions. If they listen carefully, take notes, or bring a tape recorder, your personal advocate might even remember some of the advice of the doctor or nurse a bit more clearly than you. They may help you communicate. If you find yourself getting more and more apprehensive about the needles used on you during chemotherapy treatments, your personal advocate could point out the problem to the nurse, who might suggest to the doctor that you have a port installed to save you from feeling like a human pincushion. Having a personal advocate may help you get through a time when most people are upset and confused.

The *Journal of the American Medical Association* regularly runs a column written by doctors entitled "Piece of My Mind." One contributor, Marian Block, M.D., wrote that she was horrified when an abnormality showed up on her screening mammogram. Two days later, when surgery was recommended, the thirty-nine-year-old physician experienced an "intense physiological reaction." This included feelings of fear, confusion, and disorientation, which made it suddenly difficult for the doctor to process information. "Over the next days and weeks I hear and process a lot of information, even though I am often being told facts it seems I must already know, facts with which I have an easy familiarity when they apply to others. But there are times when I am presented with information and hear almost nothing. I am like a deaf person, knowing that words are being said but unable to understand their meaning," the doctor wrote. Although her lump turned out to be benign, this experience left Dr. Block with a deeper appreciation for problems experienced by patients, and feelings strong enough to move her to write about it to other physicians. Think about it. If a doctor familiar with the terminology and processes of modern medicine can react this way to a familiar medical test and a medical procedure, it's not surprising that a layperson may not process information very well after a diagnosis of cancer. Try to compensate for what may be some very normal confusion, and bring your personal advocate to the doctor's office if you can.

Side Effects

When side effects appear, nurses follow medical protocols to mitigate them. Fortunately, even with different chemotherapy drugs, methods of treating side effects are very similar, and oncology nurses can be quite helpful in helping you cope. Since people react differently to drugs, it's understood that what works for one person may not work for the next. You may have to try a couple of antinausea medications, for instance, before you hit upon the right one to solve your particular problem. This chapter does not deal with all the physical side effects that may be experienced during chemotherapy; these are covered in chapter 11.

Receiving chemotherapy shouldn't hurt. When you receive chemotherapy treatments, you should feel no pain. If you *do* happen to feel a pain or burning sensation at the catheter or IV, notify your nurse immediately. Pain or swelling at the injection site is a sign that the needle is not positioned properly. Your catheter may have become dislodged, or medication may be leaking out of the vein into the surrounding tissues.

You should not feel nauseated during treatment. If nausea is an expected side effect of the chemotherapy, your physician should give you medication to control nausea before the treatment. Good antinausea medications such as Kytril and Zofran are proving to be very effective in relieving nausea, but it may take some experimenting to get the drugs or dosage levels just right.

If you feel nauseated, dizzy, cramped up, or uncomfortable during chemotherapy, let your nurse know exactly how you feel. The solution can be something as simple as adjusting the dosage of the medication just a bit, which your doctor might want to do. Sometimes chemotherapy drugs can be diluted with more fluid, or the rate at which you are receiving the medication can be adjusted to make you more comfortable.

It may just help relax you to watch television or listen to the radio during chemotherapy treatments. Ask your nurse if these distractions are available.

Blood Tests

Before each subsequent chemotherapy treatment, your physician will need to look at lab work such as blood test results to evaluate how you are responding to treatments. Blood tests may annoy you, but they only take a minute and they are necessary.

Blood tests provide your doctor with a quick read on how your body is responding to treatment. During chemotherapy the normal functioning of your immune system may be weakened or suppressed. Your immune system includes several types of white blood cells, including those produced in the bone marrow and the lymph nodes, which all continually circulate through your bloodstream. Chemotherapy's suppression of fast-growing white blood cells and even somewhat slow-growing red blood cells shows up dramatically in the composition of your blood after treatments. Since it takes a while for a new supply of white and red blood cells to be manufactured, a complete blood count test (CBC) may show your oncologist that the anticancer drugs are working just as expected, or that the dosage needs to be adjusted up or down.

When you receive a CBC, both white and red blood cell levels are examined. So are concentrations of blood platelets, blood cells that help your blood clot and thus seal the skin against outside infections. Platelet levels often drop during chemotherapy, with the lowest platelet counts typically coming ten to fourteen days after treatments, making your body very vulnerable to infections.

Blood cell counts frequently drop during chemotherapy. A lower than normal rate of blood cell production comes from a physical side effect known as *bone marrow suppression,* which is common with many anticancer drugs. Bone marrow suppression makes you feel weak and tired. Your blood cell levels will bounce back up, but it may take several days.

Note that your oncologist may decide to put off a chemotherapy treatment if your blood counts are low, to give your body a chance to recover its strength. This is a normal precaution and not a cause for alarm. Your treatment will be rescheduled.

If you wish to track your own progress, blood counts are an important indicator to watch. You can write this information down in your personal medical file, or graph it. Here is the normal range of cell counts that may be found in your blood:

White blood cells—4,500–11,000
Red blood cells—4.2–5.4 million in women, 4.6–6.2 million in men.
Platelets—150,000–450,000

The percentage of red blood cells or *hematocrit* ranges from 38 to 47 in women, and 40 to 54 in men.

How Doses Are Calculated

Don't be alarmed if you compare the actual doses of anticancer drugs you receive with what another person is receiving. Dosage levels can be quite different, even for people the same age with the same type of cancer. The reason is that the other person is most probably a different height and weight than you. Chemotherapy drug dosages are calculated according to body surface area (BSA). The amounts of chemotherapy drugs you receive are arrived at using this mathematical formula, which includes your height and weight.

In the doctor's office, you may also be confused by such things as temperatures recorded in degrees centigrade rather than Fahrenheit degrees, or weights expressed in kilograms rather than ounces and pounds. Remember that most of the rest of the world uses the metric system to measure almost everything, and that the metric system is the yardstick of science. These terms are only different ways of measuring familiar things, and they don't mean your height or weight has changed.

Receiving chemotherapy doesn't have to be traumatic. Although some fear and emotional confusion can be expected as you move through chemotherapy, medical treatment is more sophisticated today than it's ever been before. If you maintain a hopeful, realistic attitude about chemotherapy, you will already be a step ahead. In the next chapter, you'll learn how you can participate in the process of getting well.

9

THE EDUCATED PATIENT

How to Track and Participate in Your Own Recovery

IT IS POSSIBLE TO PARTICIPATE IN YOUR OWN RECOVERY, AND THERE is a movement underway that encourages patients to do just that. Know that you'll probably feel better about chemotherapy if you make the effort to learn about how the treatment affects you—physically and psychologically—and how you can make the demands of your treatment easier on yourself. This chapter includes suggestions about how to educate yourself, how to track your own progress, and how to open and maintain communication with your medical team.

Magazine editor Norman Cousins became a folk hero when he came down with a fatal disease and then worked to heal himself. Keeping his medical doctor informed all the way, Cousins plunged into medical literature and read everything he could about his condition. After consulting with his medical doctor, Cousins treated himself with large doses of vitamin C. He also kept himself on a steady diet of laughter by reading humorous books and watching funny movies. His miraculous recovery was the subject of a best-selling book, *Anatomy of an Illness,* which underlined the idea that, yes, patients can educate themselves and can contribute to their own recovery.

Education is a process. Educating yourself about chemotherapy involves making an effort to ask questions and to communicate your concerns. Patients may look first to the medical oncologist, and particularly the oncology nurse, to teach them about the effects of the drug or drugs they will be receiving and what kinds of experiences they might well expect.

Before chemotherapy begins, there will typically be an educational session where the doctor or the cancer nurse explains what drugs will be given and what side effects may be experienced. You may also see an educational videotape or two, and you may be given a quick tour of the hospital. You may be given printed materials relating to your treatment at this time.

If you don't receive much printed information, and if you want it, ask if more information is available. If you want more information on chemotherapy or other aspects of cancer treatment, resource groups such as the American Cancer Society will be happy to send you literature free of charge. If you haven't already done so, at this time you may want to start a file containing your medical information. Keeping your own records will help give you a feeling of control and participation in your treatment.

At this first orientation session, it's a good idea to bring along your personal advocate, another person who can sit in on the session and help you remember what is said. Your personal advocate can be your spouse, another relative, or a friend, and this person can help you speak to doctors and nurses. Your personal advocate can stand up for you, if necessary. Since you are already dealing with the chemotherapy, it may be difficult for you to remember to mention everything that concerns you to your medical team.

When coming to the doctor for tests or chemotherapy treatments, don't be afraid to bring in a "laundry list" of questions. Many doctors actually expect this, because they know there is a trend underway toward people participating in their own health care. Write all your questions down and show the list to your doctor. Be assertive. Ask your questions one at a time. If you like, bring a tape recorder. Taping any medical discussion isn't usually a problem for doctors or nurses, and listening to the tape afterward may help you remember all the details of what was said. If you have a very long list of questions, ask the receptionist to schedule a little more time with the doctor so you can be sure to get all your questions answered. Some people fax or mail their questions to the doctor in advance to save time.

These days, comprehensive cancer treatment hospitals provide patients with quite a lot of information because a lot of research has shown that well-informed patients heal faster. On the other hand, some patients are still more comfortable leaving the technical information and details to the doctors. Remember that it's perfectly all right if you don't understand *all* the technical information about chemotherapy the moment you receive it. After all, chemotherapy involves disciplines such as chemistry, microbiology, and anatomy, subjects at which you might not have excelled in school. It is perfectly all right if you don't *wish* to learn all the details of your treatment and prefer to leave those technicalities to your doctor.

Sharon Steingass, clinical director for the USC/Norris Comprehensive Cancer Center, recalls the story of a nurse who received chemotherapy. The other nurses assumed that since the patient herself was a nurse, she would want a lot of information about the anticancer drugs used in her chemotherapy. Their efforts to provide information were rebuffed. The nurse undergoing cancer treatment explained that she didn't wish to receive any information at all about the drugs she was receiving, because she wanted to be a patient this time and not a nurse.

Phone Calls

If you're receiving chemotherapy as an outpatient, you won't think of every question you wish to ask while you are sitting there in your hospital gown. Questions will come up at home or at odd times. Certainly, if your doctor orders you to call if you experience a particular side effect, make that call right away. Getting your call returned, however, may be a problem. As a general rule nurses are much easier to reach over the telephone than doctors, although some doctors are quite responsive.

When you or a family member call either a doctor or a nurse, ask whomever you speak with *when* you might expect a return

83

call. This simple little question saves you having to wait by the phone for hours and hours, if a return phone call will not be immediately forthcoming. Early on in your treatment, it's a good idea to ask if there is a preferred time to call your doctor's office with simple questions. If you have a question at an odd time, such as 3:00 A.M. on a Sunday morning, ask who you should call at that time. Alas, some doctors do not return phone calls until they have seen all the patients who have scheduled appointments. Some clinics have a particular time of day set aside for a nurse to return calls and deal with questions that come up over the course of the day. If you cannot reach someone in your doctor's office twenty-four hours a day for something like a medical emergency, find a new doctor. If you are in a health maintenance organization, call the consumer services division and make the person to whom you speak aware of your difficulties in getting your questions answered. Tell them clearly that you want a physician or a nurse to be available when you have questions that affect your health.

A footnote: Remember that when it comes to your health, there is no such thing as a stupid question. If your question is answered in medical jargon, don't be put off or intimidated. Politely ask for an explanation in language that makes sense to you. Continue to ask your question until you or your personal advocate understand what the medical professional is actually saying.

Track Your Progress

Time may seem to crawl after your treatment begins, so it may comfort you to track your own progress. Making a calendar marked with the dates scheduled for your treatments is a start. Another important thing to watch are your "tumor markers." Along with blood tests, x-ray test results, and your general physical condition, these test results provide a scientific answer to the question, How well is my treatment working?

Tumor markers are recorded as laboratory reports from tests you have been given, usually at specific intervals along your course of treatment. The actual test results to watch vary from one type of cancer to another. Some types of cancer, such as lung cancer, don't have any tumor markers.

Among the most important tumor marker test results are the prostate specific antigen (PSA) test for prostate cancer, the CA-125 test for ovarian cancer, the Beta-HCG and Alpha-Fcto protein test for testicular cancer, and the CEA test for colon cancer.

Seeing definite results from chemotherapy treatments may take some time—for colon cancer, for instance, it takes six to eight weeks of treatment and the return of results from a CAT scan. One advantage of watching these results (some methodical people even keep graphs that record their own progress) is that tracking test results helps give you a sense of control over your medical treatment and your life. You can see that something is happening to your body, because the numbers change, and you can refer back to those numbers whenever you wish. Control is something many people feel they lose during a bout with cancer, or any other chronic illness for that matter. Note that almost anything you can do to help restore your own feeling of control and continue your treatments is considered okay.

Write It Down

The best way to track your medical progress is by keeping your own personal medical file. In a special notebook, or in a file in your personal computer, you may keep a list of all the tests and treatments you receive. This file can include financial and insurance information. If there's ever a question, you'll have a record and you can look it up in a flash.

In your personal medical file, you may include the types of diagnostic tests you receive and chart their results. When and where you receive treatment may be included. The chemotherapy drugs you receive and how they are given may be recorded in your medical file, along with drugs you are given to control side effects and how well they work. You may want to keep a record of your hospitalizations, if any, including your admission and discharge dates, and your chart or unit number if you can obtain that. Marking your calendar after chemotherapy appointments may help give you the sense that your treatment has a beginning, a middle, and an end.

Billy's Story

A 67-year-old man we will call Billy has beome quite involved in his own medical care. Billy relishes the partnership he has developed with his medical team. A retired chemical engineer, Billy has received many benefits from being an educated patient who participates in the healing process.

"When I was working as an engineer, most of the work I did was as a trouble shooter. When this came along, I just turned it on myself for the first time and decided to look at the facts and work toward a solution," he says. "I'm in a better position to keep track of this data than any of the people I see. My doctors have a lot of patients, but I only have one."

Billy believes it's quite useful for patients to keep track of their own progress, as he has done by charting his blood tests results and other important medical data for critical periods over the past several years. Seeing progress on the charts and in the numbers reinforces his own sense that he is healing, he says, which strengthens his immune system.

Prior to meeting with a new doctor, Billy faxes the doctor a written summary of his medical condition, including past treatments and recent test results. He includes a list of any questions he has, and makes sure both he and the doctor have a copy when they meet face to face. This provides background information for the doctor, and saves them both time.

"After a while, doctors become quite appreciative of someone who's saving them time. I'm not asking a doctor to educate me. I'm only asking for him to give me references, and point me in the right direction," Billy says. "But doctors have to understand that you're serious, and that it doesn't just go in one ear and out the other. I make a point of writing down his answers to my questions."

Billy originally was diagnosed with prostate cancer. During the operation on his prostate, which left him with enough titanium clips in his body to set off airport metal detectors, surgeons discovered a number of enlarged lymph nodes. These turned out to be chronic lymphocyctic leukemia, which was treated with chemotherapy.

CHARTING YOUR RECOVERY

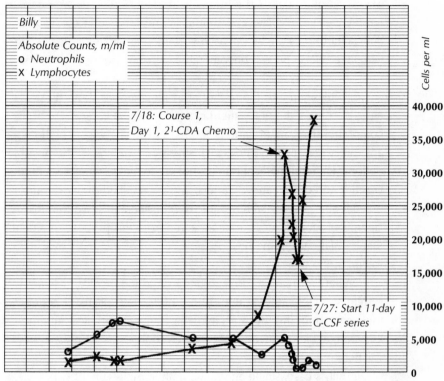

Jul. Aug. Sept. Oct. Nov. Dec. Jan. Feb. Mar. Apr. May June Jul. Aug. Sept. Oct. Nov. Dec.

Billy

Absolute Counts, m/ml
o Neutrophils
x Lymphocytes

Cells per ml

40,000

7/18: Course 1,
Day 1, 2¹-CDA Chemo

35,000

30,000

25,000

20,000

15,000

7/27: Start 11-day
G-CSF series

10,000

5,000

0

Jul. Aug. Sept. Oct. Nov. Dec. Jan. Feb. Mar. Apr. May June Jul. Aug. Sept. Oct. Nov. Dec.

1993	1994

The graph above is an actual chart made by a patient we shall call Billy, who has chronic lymphocytic leukemia. The graph tracks changes per milliliter of blood in levels of two imp-ortant types of white blood cells—lymphocytes, which were malignant, and neutrophils, which were not. The upper "o" line represents the neutrophils, and "x" line tracks lymphocytes. This graph spans one year, most of the time during which the leukemia was in remission. Neutrophil levels climbed until July, when patient received an experimental anticancer agent in a clinical trial. Neutrophil levels dropped for several weeks, until a G-CSF colony stimulating factor series began in August, creating the recovery of neutrophil levels shown at the end of the graph. Billy feels that keeping a record of important medical data helps him understand his medical condition. When he sees progress on the chart, he says, it lifts his spirits and bolsters his immune system.

Early on, Billy began keeping his own medical file containing records of his prostate specific antigen (PSA) test results, blood work, and other data. "The truth is that medical records are not terribly well kept," Billy says. "But all lab reports, studies, consultations, chart notes are available to you upon assertive request. With very little effort you can become an expert on your own data," he says.

Billy plunged into the task of educating himself about his disease, becoming the first patient to ever receive a library card at his comprehensive cancer center. Before he actually began chemotherapy, Billy spent two months exhaustively researching all the possible options. He read medical books, met with medical specialists at universities and other cancer centers, and even talked to unorthodox practitioners such as faith healers. He considers this two months "time well spent," because he emerged from this process confident that he had chosen the best possible course of treatment available to him at the time.

"What I'm trying to do is to understand the medical delivery system so that I can get the most out of it," he explains. "I get enthusiastic about this, because it increases my confidence and my knowledge. I know anything I can do to bolster my immune system will help me."

In Billy's case, single agent chemotherapy treatment with Fludaribine produced almost no side effects, and brought about a remission of the leukemia for eleven months. During this period of remission, Billy and his family, including two young grandchildren, took a month-long cross country trip, which was eventful and enjoyable. Billy also began to participate in a Wellness Community support group, something he found enormously helpful since the group's philosophy was in sync with his own efforts to particpate in his medical care.

"Anything you can do to help your immune system is an advantage in recovery," Billy says. "Using psychosocial support mechanisms like support groups just gives your immune system a chance to do its job."

After the leukemia again became aggressive, Billy elected to go into a clinical trial of an experimental anticancer agent, 2^1-CDA, which offered the rare chance of a "home run," or a complete cure of his leukemia. Unfortunately, Billy was one of the 25 percent of patients who reacted poorly to this drug. The neutrophil component of his white blood cell levels plunged—something he could clearly see on the graphs he was keeping. Because of how he felt and what he saw on his graphs, Billy refused a second treatment of the experimental drug even though his doctors urged him to try it a second time.

Before he entered the clinical trial, Billy had been using his own charts and graphs to convince his doctors that he didn't need colony stimulating factor treatments to strengthen him, since they are expensive and can have a side effect of bone pain. But when his neutrophil levels dropped after the second chemotherapy, he agreed to a G-CSF series, which was quite helpful in bringing his white blood cell levels back up to where he wanted to see them on the charts.

Billy has talked with many doctors and has some useful advice for people who wish to participate in their treatment. Do your homework, he advises, using resources like the American Cancer Society, the National Cancer Institute, and the library to educate yourself and then to work with your doctors.

"I'm not sympathetic when I hear people say their doctor won't talk to them. With some patients, it's in one ear and out the other, and doctors are busy and they don't like to waste time. Doctors have to know you're serious," Billy says, adding that physicians fear wasting time with patients who ask questions but don't actually hear or absorb their answers.

Within the medical system, Billy adds, "Assertiveness coupled with good tact is essential in dealing with medical staff. With non-medical situations such as insurance companies and the Social Security Administration, the formula seems to be more assertiveness and less tact. Written communcation is at least an order of magnitude more effective than oral presentation," he says.

Billy firmly believes that men and women ought to participate in their own health care both by educating themselves and by participating in support groups.

"When you get cancer, you just have two choices. Many people simply prepare to die. But a lot of us luckier ones prepare to live. For some of us, it takes that kind of wake-up call," Billy adds. "Right now, I think every relationship of mine has improved, some by being strengthened, some by being terminated. I don't have time for that negative stuff anymore."

Mary-Ellen Siegel, author of *The Cancer Patient's Handbook*, suggests that you give your physician a personal contact list for placement with your medical chart. This list would include your next of kin or someone you consider your next of kin, people who may give you emotional support, and people the doctor has your permission to discuss your medical condition with (and those whom you *don't want* to know the specifics of your medical condition). Be sure you include full names, addresses, and telephone numbers where appropriate, and specify where or when they might be needed.

Your medical file might also include important phone numbers—your medical oncologist, family doctor, dentist, nurse, pharmacist, ambulance company, as well as important family members and neighbors.

Keeping a personal medical file, or even a personal diary, can help give you back a sense of control over your own life. Some large cancer centers like the USC/Norris Comprehensive Cancer Center actually give patients an attractive personal notebook and encourage them to use it as a personal journal or record-keeping device. The notebook includes a page of plastic slipcovers to hold business cards from medical specialists, and many other features including blank pages on which patients may write medical information, or anything they wish.

Many people find it comforting to keep a personal journal, writing down anything they wish to express about their lives, their dreams, and any other thoughts or observations they wish to remember. Keeping a diary might have health benefits. Studies at

Southern Methodist University have measured the differences in immune system function between people who wrote about their traumatic experiences in a diary versus people who did not write them down. The people who wrote about their trauma in diaries actually had better blood tests for immune function, and made fewer visits to the doctor during the time of the study than the control group.

One of the best ways to participate in your treatment is by educating yourself in any way you can. Read and learn about your disease and its treatment, as you are doing at this moment by reading this book.

"After I was first diagnosed with cancer, my friends would give me articles to read, but I read everything negative into them," one woman confessed after she recovered from cancer. She added that as her psychological outlook improved, so did her ability to rationally process information.

Many worthwhile books have been written on various aspects of cancer. One of the very best sourcebooks on all types of cancer therapy is *Everyone's Guide to Cancer Therapy,* edited by Malin Dollinger, M.D., a sort of encyclopedia of cancer treatment first published in 1991. Dr. Dollinger's book is a good place to begin reading about the medical aspects of cancer in greater depth, including the recommended treatments at various stages of cancer. Several other good books are listed in the Other Resources appendix of this book.

Local libraries and bookstores often have an excellent selection of health-related books. Many college and university medical libraries may have on-line reference catalogs such as MEDLINE, which list books and magazine articles written about different aspects of cancer treatment. Reference librarians can be enormously helpful in locating information on particular topics.

More and more information is available through the Internet and computer on-line services, which may be accessed from your home with a personal computer. Computer chat groups discuss medical subjects of interest, as do professional forums comprised mostly of medical professionals. As is discussed later, these chats in cyberspace are not always an accurate source of medical information, but they can be. Some medical information is available in interactive formats such as CD-ROM.

Information is printed in books, in magazines, or in pamphlet form. Information comes to you in conversations with other people, from radio and television, from your telephone line, or from your computer screen. With any medical information you hear or receive, always consider the source.

Educating yourself can be important, but move at your own speed. Accumulating information about what is occurring during chemotherapy will help you survive the process, which after all does have a beginning, a middle, and an end.

Since all chemotherapy treatments involve chemotherapy drugs, the next chapter includes a comprehensive listing of the most commonly used anticancer agents and their most common physical side effects. Look at this chapter, and the chapters that follow, as steps forward in your education.

10

ANTICANCER DRUGS

A SURVEY OF THE FIFTY-SEVEN MOST COMMONLY USED ANTICANCER AGENTS AND THEIR MOST COMMON SIDE EFFECTS

THIS CHAPTER PROBABLY CONTAINS INFORMATION ON THE CHEMOTHERAPY drugs being used in your treatment. It includes a listing of the major drug groups and an explanation of how they work, plus a survey of the fifty-seven most commonly used anticancer agents and their most common side effects. By learning about the drugs used in your treatment, and what side effects you can expect, you will be better prepared to handle chemotherapy and further educate yourself.

By now you realize that medical oncologists have a great variety of anticancer agents at their disposal. Many are given in particular combinations designed to attack cancer cells at different stages of their growth cycle. Some are biologic agents that occur in nature, such as derivatives of the periwinkle plant or certain bacteria. A few, like hormones and steroids, are substances that are produced in the human body. Most are chemical drugs that do not occur in a state of nature.

The major groups of anticancer drugs include:

Alkylating agents such as nitrogen mustard, carboplatin, and cis-platin block reproduction of the chain of cancer cell DNA during cell division. They may be used in the treatment of several cancers including breast and lung cancer, and some leukemias and lymphomas.

Antimetabolites such as fluorouracil and methotrexate cause cancer cells to die by preventing the production of proteins and nucleic acids that cancer cells need to form their DNA. They are called "counterfeit molecules," because they fool cancer cells into accepting them, but this leads to the formation of defective DNA, which breaks the normal growth cycle of cancerous cells. They may be used to treat the leukemias, breast, colon, pancreatic, and other cancers.

Tumoricidal antibiotics such as doxorubicin (Adriamycin) and bleomycin interfere with various functions of the cancerous cell and may inhibit DNA, RNA, or protein synthesis. Made from substances that occur in nature such as fungi in the soil, these antibiotics are so powerful and toxic that they are not normally used against bacterial infections like most antibiotics. May be used to treat Hodgkin's disease, cervical, testicular, breast, bladder, thyroid, and other cancers.

Other chemotherapy drugs include steroid hormones, enzymes, and mitotic inhibitors:

Steroid hormones are hormones such as the androgens (testosterone), which change the balance of hormones necessary for the growth of tumors. They may be used against breast and uterine cancer, multiple myeloma, Hodgkin's disease, leukemias, and lymphomas.

Enzymes such as asparaginase break down amino acids necessary for cancer cell growth. Enzymes and other anticancer drugs that don't fit into the above categories may be used against leukemias, bladder, lung, ovarian, and other cancers.

Mitotic inhibitors such as vinblastine and vincristine are natural substances derived from the periwinkle plant, which stop cancer cells from dividing normally. They may be used against cancers such as Hodgkin's disease, choriocarcinoma, breast cancer, lung cancer, testicular cancer, neuroblastoma, and acute lymphocytic leukemia.

Side Effects

Some anticancer drugs happily produce few or no side effects in most patients. On the other hand, some very annoying side effects are fairly predictable with certain chemotherapy drugs, even though many expected side effects may be controlled by methods such as those listed in the following chapter.

You should understand that your reaction to chemotherapy will be individual and based on many factors, including your general health, age and body chemistry, the stage of the disease, the type of cancer, which chemotherapy drugs are administered, and more. Your mental state is important, too, because your emotional state can either intensify or mitigate the side effects you experience.

Although he or she may be quite bright, your oncologist does not have a crystal ball and therefore cannot predict all the side effects you will experience. More than likely your oncologist will relay the available statistical information about probable side effects, and make some observations based on his or her own experience. Understand that doctors don't know exactly what you'll experience. Although they have been trained in the scientific method, many doctors prefer to err on the side of caution. Remember that most people find chemotherapy to be a less traumatic experience than they expect.

Anticancer Drugs

What follows is a list of the fifty-seven most commonly used anticancer agents as compiled by the National Cancer Institute (NCI). These are listed alphabetically by generic name, with listings that include each drug's most common other names or brand names, which in a couple of cases were too numerous to list.

Listings include the type or class of drug, the method of administration, the types of cancer for which a particular drug is typically used, and the more common side effects, as well as side effects that should be reported to your doctor immediately. Much of the following information is taken from the National Cancer Institute's fact sheets on specific medications, which are available free of charge by calling the NCI's toll-free telephone number listed in the Other Resources appendix of this book. This data is supplemented in a few cases with more detailed information from the PDQ database and National Cancer Society publications.

This list is *not* intended as medical advice. Medical advice should always come from your oncologist. Whether they're listed here or not, any side effects you experience that concern you should *always* be reported to your doctor, the undisputed expert on these matters. Don't worry that you're imposing by talking about your side effects, even if they seem minor or unimportant, because the information you communicate to your doctor or cancer nurse can be used to make your chemotherapy more effective.

Only the most common side effects are listed below. This list is not intended to be a complete summary of all possible side effects that may be experienced. Always consult with your doctor regarding possible side effects of any medication.

The Fifty-Seven Most Commonly Used Anti-Cancer Drugs

1. **Altretamine,** brand names include Hexalen, Hexastat, and hexamethylmelamine. An alkylating agent, administered orally. Used to treat cancer of the ovaries. Side effects, which should be reported to your doctor, include anxiety, clumsiness, confusion, dizziness, mental depression, numbness in limbs, and weakness. More common side effects include nausea and vomiting.

2. **Aminoglutethimide,** brand name Cytadren. An antihormonal agent, administered orally. Used to treat breast, prostate, and adrenal cancer. More common side effects include clumsiness, dizziness or lightheadedness when standing up, drowsiness,

lack of energy, loss of appetite, skin rash or itching, nausea, and uncontrolled eye movements.

3. **Androgens,** generic names include fluoxymesterone, methyitestosterone, testosterone, testosterone cypionate, testosterone enanthate, and testosterone priopionate. More than forty brand names exist for the androgens, so check with your pharmacist, doctor, or nurse for the name of your drug. Androgens are male hormones, administered orally. Used to treat breast cancer in females, and for some other conditions. For females, the most common side effects, which should be reported to your doctor, include acne or oily skin, enlarged clitoris, hair loss, deepening of voice, irregular periods, and unnatural hair growth. For males, the most common side effects, which should be reported to your doctor, include acne, breast soreness, frequent erections, frequent urge to urinate, and increased breast size.

4. **Asparaginase,** other names include Elspar, l-asparaginase, and colaspase. An enzyme, administered by injection. Used to treat some types of cancer including acute lymphoblastic leukemia, and lymphomas. Side effects, which should be reported to your doctor immediately, include joint pain, puffy face, skin rash or itch, stomach pain accompanied by nausea and vomiting, and trouble breathing. More common side effects include headache, loss of appetite, nausea or vomiting, stomach cramps, and weight loss.

5. **Bacillus Calmette-Guerin,** brand names include TheraCys and TICE BCG. A biologic agent, administered mucosal-local. Used to treat bladder cancer. Side effects, which should be reported to your doctor immediately, include blood in urine, fever and chills, frequent urge to urinate, more frequent urination, joint pain, nausea and vomiting, and a severe or continuing painful urination. Other more common side effects can include a burning sensation during the first urination after treatment.

6. **Bleomycin,** brand name Blenoxane. An antitumor antibiotic, administered by injection. Used to treat some types of cancer

including squamous carcinoma of the head and neck, Hodgkin's and non-Hodgkin's lymphoma, testes, anus, vulva, uterus, cervix, and malignant pleural effusions. Side effects, which should be reported to your doctor immediately, are chills and fever within three to six hours after a chemotherapy treatment. More common side effects, which should also be reported to your doctor, are cough, shortness of breath, and sores in mouth or on lips. Other common side effects are skin darkening, mouth and intestinal ulcers, lung scarring, fever, allergic reactions such as itching or skin rash, swelling of fingers, vomiting, and loss of appetite.

7. **Busulfan,** brand name Myleran. An alkylating agent, administered orally. Used to treat some types of cancer including chronic myelogenous leukemia, and in bone marrow transplantation. Side effects, which should be reported to your doctor, include black, tarry stools, blood in urine or defecation, pinpoint-sized red spots on skin, and unusual bleeding or bruising. More common side effects include darkening of the skin and irregular menstruation for women. The most common side effect is bone marrow suppression.

8. **Carboplatin,** brand name Paraplatin. An alkylating-like agent, administered by injection. Used to treat some types of cancer including ovarian, cervical, small cell lung, head and neck, bladder, testes, mesothelioma, and brain cancer. Most common side effects include nausea or vomiting, unusual tiredness, weakness, and fatigue.

9. **Carmustine,** other names include BiCNU and BCNU. Administered by injection. Used to treat some types of cancer including brain, Hodgkin's disease, lymphomas, myeloma, melanoma, and lung cancer. A side effect, which should be reported to your doctor, is shortness of breath, which may be more likely if you smoke. Most common side effects are prolonged bone marrow suppression, nausea, and vomiting.

10. **Chlorambucil,** brand name Leukeran. An alkylating agent, administered orally. Used to treat some types of cancer including chronic lymphatic leukemia, Hodgkin's and non-

Hodgkin's lymphoma, breast and ovarian cancer, and for other conditions. Side effects, which should be reported to your doctor immediately, include sores in mouth or on lips. Most common side effects are bone marrow suppression and mild nausea. Sometimes causes hair loss.

11. **Cisplatin,** brand names include Platinol and Platinol-AQ. An alkylating-like agent, administered by injection. Used to treat some types of cancer including testes, ovarian, head and neck, Hodgkin's and non-Hodgkin's lymphoma, sarcomas, bladder, lung, stomach, cervix, myeloma, prostate, and mesothelioma. Common side effects, which should be reported to your doctor immediately, include joint pain, loss of balance, lower back pain or side pain, ringing in ears, swelling of feet or lower legs, trouble hearing, and unusual fatigue. More common side effects include nausea and vomiting, sometimes severe.

12. **Cyclophosphamide,** brand names include Cytoxan and NEOSAR. An alkylating agent, administered orally or by injection. Used to treat some types of cancer including Hodgkin's and non-Hodgkin's lymphoma, multiple myeloma, sarcomas, leukemia, neuroblastoma, breast, lung, testes, endometrium, mycosis fungoides cancer, and kidney disease. Side effects, which should be reported to your doctor, include dizziness, confusion or agitation, unusual fatigue, and missing menstrual periods. More common side effects include bone marrow suppression, hair loss, darkening of skin or fingernails, loss of appetite, nausea, and vomiting.

13. **Cyclosporine,** brand names include Sandimmune, ciciosporin, and Cyclosporine A. An immunosuppressive agent, administered orally. Used to prevent the body from rejecting the transplant of organs such as kidney, liver, or heart transplant. Side effects, which should be reported to your doctor, include tender, swollen, or bleeding gums. Some more common side effects include increase in the growth of hair and trembling or shaking of hands.

14. **Cytarabine,** or cytosine arabinoside, brand names include Cytosar-U and Ara-C. An antimetabolite, administered by in-

jection. Used to treat some types of cancers including acute leukemia, lymphoma, head and neck cancer. Side effects, which should be reported to your doctor, include sores in mouth or on lips. More common side effects include bone marrow suppression, nausea, vomiting, and diarrhea.

15. **Dacarbazine,** or DTIC-Dome. An alkylating agent, administered by injection. Used to treat some types of cancers including Hodgkin's disease, malignant melanoma, sarcomas, carcinoid, islet cell and medullary thyroid cancer. Side effects, which should be reported to your doctor immediately, include redness, pain, or swelling at the place of injection. Most common side effects include bone marrow suppression, nausea, and vomiting.

16. **Dactinomycin,** or Cosmegen or Actinomycin-D. An antitumor antibiotic, administered by injection. Used to treat some types of cancers including testes, melanoma, choriocarcinoma, Wilms' tumor, neuroblastoma, retinoblastoma, Kaposi's sarcoma, and sarcomas. Side effects, which should be reported to your doctor, include continuing diarrhea, difficulty in swallowing, heartburn, continuing stomach pain, and sores in mouth or on lips. More common side effects are darkening or redness of skin, skin rash, fatigue, nausea, and vomiting.

17. **Daunorubicin,** or Cerubidine. An antitumor antibiotic, administered by injection. Used to treat some types of cancer including acute lymphoblastic and myelogenous leukemia. Side effects, which should be reported to your doctor, include sores in mouth and on lips. Most common side effects are bone marrow suppression, nausea, vomiting, and hair loss. Red urine is expected for a day or two after chemotherapy treatment.

18. **Doxorubicin,** or Adriamycin PFS, Adriamycin RDF, or Rubex. An antitumor antibiotic, administered by injection. Used to treat some types of cancers including lung, breast, bladder, prostate, pancreas, stomach, ovary, thyroid, endometrium, sarcoma, leukemia, Hodgkin's and non-Hodgkin's lymphoma, mesothelioma myeloma, Wilms' tumor and cancer of unknown primary site. Side effects, which should be reported to

your doctor, include sores in mouth or on lips. Most common side effects include nausea and vomiting and loss of hair. Urine will turn red in color for one to two days after treatment.

19. **Estradiol,** or Estraderm. A hormonal agent, administered through patches placed on the skin. Provides additional hormones after certain types of surgery in females, and for other conditions. Side effects, which should be reported to your doctor, include breast pain, increased breast size, swelling of feet or lower legs, and rapid weight gain. More common side effects include bloating of stomach, cramps, loss of appetite, nausea, skin irritation, and redness on site of patch.

20. **Estramustine,** or Emcyt. An antihormonal agent, administered orally. Used to treat some cases of prostate cancer. Side effects, which should be reported to your doctor, include swelling of feet or lower legs. More common side effects include breast tenderness or enlargement, decreased interest in sex, diarrhea, and nausea.

21. **Estrogens (IV).** Generic names include chlorotrianisene, diethylstilbestrol, estradiol, estrogens, estrone, estropipate, ethinyl estradiol, and quinestrol. More than sixty brand names exist for estrogens—consult your pharmacist, doctor, or nurse for the name of your drug. A female hormone, administered by injection. Used to treat some cases of breast cancer in men or women, prostate cancer, to provide additional hormones after surgery, and for other conditions. Side effects, which should be reported to your doctor, include breast pain, increased breast size, and swelling of feet and lower legs. Another side effect for women who have not had their uterus removed and are taking estrogen in combination with the female hormone progestin is that they may begin having monthly vaginal bleeding similar to menstruation.

22. **Estrogens (oral).** More than sixty brand names and generic names (see number 21). A female hormone, administered orally. Used to treat some cases of breast cancer in men or women, prostate cancer, to provide additional hormones after surgery, and for other conditions. Side effects are similar to es-

trogens in number 21, with the addition of nausea and vomiting, which are more common.

23. **Etoposide (IV),** or VePesid or VP-16. A plant alkaloid, administered by injection. Used primarily for testes cancer, some types of lung cancer, acute nonlymphocytic leukemia, lymphoma, and head and neck cancer. Most common side effects include bone marrow suppression, loss of appetite, loss of hair, nausea, and vomiting.
24. **Etoposide (oral),** or VePesid or VP-16. A plant alkaloid, administered orally. Used to treat some types of lung cancer and occasionally some other types of cancer. Side effects similar to number 23.
25. **Floxuridine,** or FUDR. An antimetabolite, administered by injection. Used to treat some types of cancer including cancer of the liver and head and neck cancer. Side effects, which should be reported to your doctor immediately, include diarrhea, sores in mouth or on lips, and stomach pain or cramps. Sometimes causes loss of hair.
26. **Fluorouracil,** or Adrucil or 5-FU. An antimetabolite, administered by injection. Used to treat some types of cancer including breast, stomach, colon, liver, pancreas, ovarian, bladder, and prostate cancer. Can be used topically for skin cancer. Side effects, which should be reported to your doctor immediately, include diarrhea, heartburn, and sores in mouth and on lips. More common side effects include bone marrow suppression, loss of appetite, nausea and vomiting, skin rash or itching, loss of hair, and fatigue.
27. **Flutamide,** or Eulexin. An antihormonal/antiandrogen agent, administered orally. Used in some cases of prostate cancer. More common side effects include decreased sexual desire, diarrhea, impotence, nausea or vomiting, and hot flashes (sudden sweating or feelings of warmth).
28. **Goserelin,** or Zoladex. A hormonal agent, administered by injection. Used in some cases of prostate cancer. More common side effects include decrease in sexual desire, impotence, and sudden sweating or hot flashes.

29. **Hydroxyurea** or Hydrea. An antimetabolite, administered orally. Used to treat some types of cancer including chronic myelogenous leukemia, head and neck, kidney, brain, melanoma, and ovarian cancer. Most common side effect is bone marrow suppression. Other side effects include diarrhea, drowsiness, loss of appetite, nausea, and vomiting.

30. **Ifosfamide,** or IFEX. An alkylating agent, administered by injection. Used to treat cancer of the testes, non-Hodgkin's lymphoma, lung, ovarian, sarcomas, melanoma, and chronic lymphocytic leukemia. Side effects, which should be reported to your doctor immediately, include confusion, hallucinations, blood in urine, and frequent or painful urination. More common side effects, which should also be reported to your doctor, include unusual fatigue or tiredness. Other common side effects include nausea or vomiting, and sometimes loss of hair.

31. **Interferons,** Alpha, or Alferon N, Intron A, or Roferon-A. A biologic agent, administered by injection. Used to treat hairy cell leukemia, Kaposi's sarcoma (AIDS-related), melanoma, kidney, myeloma, chronic myelogenous leukemia, and lymphoma. More common side effects include aching muscles, change in taste/metallic taste of food, chills and fever during the first week or two of treatment, general feeling of discomfort or illness, headache, loss of appetite, nausea and vomiting, skin rash, and unusual fatigue.

32. **Interleukin-2,** or Aldesleukin, IL-2, or Proleukin. A biologic agent, administered by injection. Used to treat cancer of the kidney. Side effects, which should be reported to your doctor immediately, include fever or chills and shortness of breath. Common side effects, which should also be reported to your doctor, include agitation, confusion, diarrhea, dizziness, drowsiness, mental depression, nausea, and vomiting, sores in mouth or on lips, tingling of hands or feet, unusual decrease in urination, unusual tiredness, or weight gain of five to ten pounds or more. Your doctor will also want to watch for anemia, heart problems, kidney problems, liver problems, low blood pressure, low platelet counts or low white blood cell counts, and underactive thyroid. Other common side effects include dry

skin, loss of appetite, skin rash or redness with burning or itching followed by peeling,unusual discomfort, and illness.

33. **Leucovorin,** or Wellcovorin, folinic acid, citrovorum factor, or leucovorin calcium. A protecting agent, administered orally or by injection. Used as an antidote to some anticancer drugs such as methotrexate, or a potentiating agent when used with fluorouracil. Also prevents or treats certain types of anemia. Side effects, which should be reported to your doctor immediately, include skin rash, hives, itching, and wheezing.

34. **Leuprolide,** or Lupron or Lupron Depot. A hormonal agent, administered by injection. Used to treat cancer of the prostate, and for other conditions. More common side effects include decrease in sexual desire or impotence, nausea or vomiting, and sudden sweats or hot flashes.

35. **Levamisole,** or Ergamisol. An immunomodulating agent frequently used with fluorouracil to treat colon cancer, administered orally. More common side effects include diarrhea, metallic taste, and nausea.

36. **Lomustine,** or CeeNu or CCNU. An alkylating agent, administered orally. Used to treat some types of cancer including Hodgkin's and non-Hodgkin's lymphoma, brain, melanoma, kidney, and lung cancer. Most common side effects are prolonged bone marrow suppression, nausea, vomiting, and sometimes loss of hair.

37. **Mechlorethamine,** or mustargen or nitrogen mustard. An alkylating agent, administered by injection. Used to treat some types of cancer including Hodgkin's and non-Hodgkin's lymphoma, malignant pleural effusions, lung, and mycosis fungoides. Side effects, which should be reported to your doctor, include missing menstrual periods and painful rash. Most common side effects are bone marrow suppression, nausea, vomiting, and sometimes loss of hair.

38. **Melphalan,** or Alkeran, L-PAM, or phenylalanine mustard. An alkylating agent, administered orally. Used to treat multiple myeloma, ovarian, and breast cancer. Most common side ef-

fects are bone marrow suppression and occasionally nausea or vomiting.

39. **Mercaptopurine,** or Purinethol, or 6-MP. An antimetabolite, administered orally. Used to treat some types of cancer including acute leukemia, chronic myelogenous leukemia, and immunosuppression. Side effects, which should be reported to your doctor, include unusual fatigue, and yellow eyes or skin. Most common side effects include bone marrow suppression and sometimes loss of hair.

40. **Mesna,** or Mesnex. Administered by injection. A protecting agent used to reduce harmful effects on the bladder from the effects of some chemotherapy drugs such as ifosfamide and Cytoxan in high dosages.

41. **Methotrexate,** or Folex, Folex PFS, Mexate, Mexate-AQ, Rheumatrex, or amethopterin. An antimetabolite, administered orally or by injection. Used to treat some types of cancer including acute leukemia, sarcoma, choriocarcinoma, head and neck, breast, lung, stomach, esophagus, testes, lymphoma, and mycosis fungoides. Side effects, which should be reported to your doctor immediately, include black, tarry stools, bloody vomit, diarrhea, reddening of skin, sores in mouth or on lips, and stomach pain. Most common side effects include bone marrow suppression, nausea, and vomiting.

42. **Mitomycin**, or Mutamycin. An alkylating agent, administered by injection. Used to treat some types of cancers including colon, stomach, pancreas, esophagus, anus, breast, lung, cervix, and bladder cancer. Most common side effects include bone marrow suppression, nausea, vomiting, loss of appetite, and sometimes loss of hair.

43. **Mitotane,** or Lysodren or o,p'-DDD. An antihormonal agent, administered orally. Used to treat cancer of the adrenal cortex. Side effects, which should be reported to your doctor, include darkening of skin, diarrhea, dizziness, drowsiness, loss of appetite, mental depression, nausea and vomiting, skin rash, and unusual fatigue.

44. **Mitoxantrone,** or Novantrone. An antitumor antibiotic, administered by injection. Used to treat some types of cancer including acute leukemia, breast, ovarian, and lymphomas. Side effects, which should be reported to your doctor immediately, include black, tarry stools, coughing, and shortness of breath. Another side effect, which should be reported to your doctor, is stomach pain. More common side effects include diarrhea, headaches, nausea, and vomiting.

45. **Plicamycin,** or Mithracin or mithramycin. An antitumor antibiotic, administered by injection. Used to treat some types of cancer, and to treat the condition *hypercalcemia* (too much calcium in the blood), which occurs with some types of cancers. *Signs of overdose,* which should be reported to your doctor immediately, include bloody or black, tarry stools, flushing or redness or swelling in face, nosebleed, skin rash, sore throat and fever, unusual bleeding or bruising, and vomiting of blood. Other more common side effects include diarrhea, irritation or soreness of mouth, loss of appetite, nausea, and vomiting.

46. **Prednisone,** or Apr-Prednisone, Deltasone, Liquid Pred, Meticorten, Orasone 1, Orasone 5, Orasone 10, Orasone 20, Orasone 50, Prednicen-M, Prednisone Intensol, Sterapred, Sterapred DS, or Winpred. An adrenocorticoid or hormonal agent which is administered orally. Used to treat acute and chronic lymphocytic leukemia, Hodgkin's and non-Hodgkin's lymphoma, myeloma, breast, and brain metastases, as well as some noncancerous conditions. Common side effects include increased appetite, indigestion, nervousness, restlessness, and trouble sleeping. Side effects, which should be reported to your doctor *with long-term use,* include back or rib pain, bloody or black stools, chronic stomach pain or burning, puffiness in face, irregular heartbeats, menstrual problems, muscle cramps, pain, fatigue, reddish purple lines on skin, swelling of feet, thin or shiny skin, and rapid weight gain.

47. **Procarbazine,** or Matulane. An alkylating agent, administered orally. Used to treat some types of cancer such as brain cancer. Side effects, which should be reported to your doctor, include

confusion, convulsions, cough, hallucinations, missing periods, shortness of breath, thickening of bronchial secretions, and continuing fatigue or weakness. More common side effects include drowsiness, pain in joints, muscle pain or twitching, nausea or vomiting, nervousness, nightmares, trouble sleeping, unusual fatigue, and weakness.

48. **Progestins,** or progestinal agents, known by several other names including Amen, Aygestin, Curretab, Cycrin, Delalutin, Depo-Provera, Duralutin, Femotrone, Gesterol L.A., Hylutin, Hyprogest, Hyproval P.A., Megace, Micronor, Norethisterone, Norlutate, Norlutin, Nor-QD, Ovrette, Pro-Depo, Prodrox, Progestaject, Progestilin, and Provera. A hormonal agent, administered orally. Used to treat breast, prostate, uterine, and kidney cancer. These side effects are rare with this drug, but you should immediately get emergency help if you experience a sudden or severe headache, loss of coordination, loss or change in vision, shortness of breath or slurred speech, pains in chest, groin, or leg, unusual weakness, numbness, and pain in arm or leg. A more common side effect is a change in the menstrual cycle, which should be reported to your doctor. More common side effects include changes in appetite, changes in weight, swelling of ankles and feet, unusual tiredness, and weakness.

49. **Streptozocin,** or Zanosar. An alkylating agent, administered by injection. Used to treat some types of cancer such as cancer of the pancreas. Side effects, which should be reported to your doctor, include swelling of feet or lower legs and unusual decrease in urination. Most common side effects include nausea and vomiting.

50. **Tamoxifen,** or Nolvadex, Novadex-D, or tamoxifen citrate. An antihormonal agent, administered orally. Used to treat some cases of breast cancer, endometrium, and ovarian cancer. More common side effects include hot flashes, nausea or vomiting, and weight gain.

52. **Taxol,** or Paclitaxel. An antineoplastic, administered by injectionl. Used to treat cancers such as cancer of the breast or

ovary. Side effects, which should be reported to your doctor immediately, include cough or harshness, fever or chills, lower back or side pain, and painful or difficult urination. More common side effects, which should also be reported to your doctor, include flushing of face, shortness of breath, and skin rash or itching. Other common side effects your doctor will watch for include anemia and low white blood cell or platelet counts. Other more common side effects include diarrhea, nausea and vomiting, numbness, burning, tingling in hands or feet, and pain in joints or muscles such as arms or legs beginning two to three days after treatment, which can last as long as five days.

52. **Testolactone,** or Teslac. A hormonal agent, administered orally. Used to treat some cases of breast cancer in females. Infrequently causes diarrhea, loss of appetite, nausea or vomiting, pain in lower extremities, rash, and swelling or redness of tongue.

53. **Thioguanine,** or Tabloid. An antimetabolite, administered orally or injected. Used to treat some types of cancer such as acute nonlymphocytic leukemia. Most common side effects are bone marrow suppression, occasionally loss of appetite, diarrhea, nausea, and skin rash.

54. **Thiotepa,** or triethylenethiophosphoramide. An alkylating agent, administered by injection. Used to treat some types of cancer such as breast, bladder, ovarian, Hodgkin's disease, and bone marrow transplantation. Most common side effect is bone marrow suppression.

55. **Uracil Mustard.** An alkylating agent, administered orally. Used to treat some types of cancer. More common side effects include diarrhea, nausea, and vomiting.

56. **Vinblastine,** or Velban, Velsar, or vinblastine sulfate. A plant alkaloid, administered by injection. Used to treat some types of cancer such as Hodgkin's disease, choriocarcinoma, testes, breast, lung, and Kaposi's sarcoma. Most common side effects include bone marrow suppression, nausea, vomiting, constipation, and sometimes loss of hair. Can cause burns if it leaks out of the vein.

57. **Vincristine,** or Oncovin, Vincasar PFS, Vincrez, or vincristine sulfate. A plant alkaloid, administered by injection. Used to treat some types of cancer including acute lymphocytic leukemia, Hodgkin's and non-Hodgkin's lymphoma, neuroblastoma, testes, sarcomas, lung, breast, cervical cancer, and Wilms' tumor. Side effects, which should be reported to your doctor, include blurred or double vision, constipation, difficulty walking, drooping eyelids, headache, jaw pain, joint pain, lower back or side pain, numbness or tingling in fingers and toes, pain in fingers and toes, pain in testicles, stomach cramps, swelling of feet or lower legs, and weakness. Can cause loss of hair.

Although you won't experience every possible side effect, you may well experience a few. The next chapter explains some ways to deal with the side effects you may experience, and to make your chemotherapy treatments more manageable.

11

PHYSICAL SIDE EFFECTS

SOME WAYS TO HELP YOU MITIGATE THEIR EFFECTS

THIS CHAPTER DEALS WITH THE PHYSICAL SIDE EFFECTS OF CHEMOTHERAPY, which can be quite powerful although they are almost always transitory. More than a dozen of the most common physical side effects experienced from chemotherapy drugs are included here, with suggestions on how to relieve them. Keep in mind that no one experiences all these side effects.

Methods and techniques to manage side effects include medications available to you through your doctor, practical or behavioral changes, and dietary and nutritional modifications that are helpful with some side effects, such as diarrhea. Nutritional methods of relieving some side effects are included in this chapter as a matter of convenience rather than in chapter 12, which deals with diet and nutrition, because the aim was to bundle this information in a central location that could be easily accessed and applied. Not included here are psychological or social side effects such as emotional stress, which are dealt with in later chapters.

Remember, no one experiences *all* the possible physical side effects of chemotherapy. More and more people undergoing chemotherapy experience no side effects at all, or side effects that are mild and easily controlled. Certainly, any side effects that are unusual or that bother you should be reported to your physician.

Your medical oncologist is the final authority on controlling the physical side effects of chemotherapy.

Why Side Effects Occur

Your entire bloodstream may be flooded with powerful toxins for a short time during chemotherapy treatments, and many anticancer drugs pack quite a wallop. Chemotherapy's short, powerful toxic rush affects all of your body, especially those groups of cells whose rapid growth rates are similar to the growth rates of cancer cells, which the anticancer agents seek to destroy.

Cells grow and divide quickly in the hair follicles, which is the reason why you need to periodically cut your hair. Some of your fastest growing cells keep your skin smooth and your fingernails hard, forcing you to get a manicure now and then. Cells are continually produced and sluffed off all along the gastrointestinal system, which begins at your mouth and ends at your rectum, and includes the esophagus, stomach, and intestines. The cell growth and destruction that occurs inside your gastrointestinal system is a part of the complex natural process that routinely breaks down and digests an overwhelming variety of plant or animal foods. Within your bone marrow, a fresh new supply of nascent red and white blood cells called "stem cells" is constantly and quickly being generated. Within your body, approximately ten milllion cells are replaced every second.

Physical side effects spring from chemotherapy's inadvertent poisoning of these fast-growing cell groups, and the temporary knockdown of these cell populations that a dose of toxic chemicals imposes on your body. Most physical side effects are quite temporary, although in a few cases heart, lung, or reproductive organ damage can remain after treatment, and other side effects may occur years after treatment. Most side effects will eventually pass due to your body's extraordinary ability to heal and mend itself over time. Side effects are evidence that the chemotherapy drugs are affecting your body, and an unpleasant reminder that the drugs are working.

Physical side effects include *immediate* side effects that can come and go soon after the chemotherapy treatment is completed, such as nausea or vomiting. *Chronic* side effects such as low blood counts may linger through the course of treatment and sometimes beyond.

Achieving Control

Utilizing a multidisciplinary approach to the side effects of chemotherapy allows you to attack the physical symptoms you experience from several angles, some of which you control. You may find that combination of medical and nonmedical techniques that is most effective for you in mitigating the side effects you experience. For example, one side effect, which has obvious psychological and physical elements, is pain, which chapter 14 discusses. Pain may be relieved by medical means, of course, but for many people some pain relief can be achieved, or the effects of medicine enhanced, by the employment of self-help, stress-relieving exercises and techniques such as those listed in chapter 16.

The following list of physical side effects may be intimidating if you have not yet begun chemotherapy treatment. Please remember—nobody ever experiences *all* the possible medical side effects of chemotherapy. Your doctor will give you an idea of what side effects you might reasonably expect from chemotherapy. However, as you've probably discovered by now, it does no harm to be prepared.

Common Side Effects

Here is a list of the most common physical side effects of chemotherapy:

- Nausea
- Hair loss
- Loss of appetite
- Fatigue or anemia
- Infection

- Blood clotting problems
- Mouth, gum, and throat problems
- Diarrhea
- Constipation
- Nerve and muscle effects
- Skin and nail changes
- Kidney and bladder effects
- Fluid retention
- Tooth decay
- Sexual/reproductive changes

Nausea and Vomiting

Chemotherapy drugs can affect either the stomach itself, or the part of the brain that controls the impulse to vomit. People who experience the side effects of nausea or vomiting can feel a bit nauseous most of the time, or very nauseous only part of the time. Nausea frequently begins a few hours after chemotherapy treatment, and some people may feel nauseated for a day or two. In addition, some people experience anticipatory nausea, in which they begin to vomit before their actual treatment begins. One medical oncologist tells the story of a patient he ran into in the supermarket many years after chemotherapy—the patient recognized the doctor, paused to say hello, and then vomited.

Chemotherapy drugs that frequently cause nausea include cisplatin, cyclophosphamide, dacarbazine, dactinomycin, mechlorethamine, and streptozocin. Chemotherapy drugs with a *low* potential for creating nausea include bleomycin, fluorouracil, etoposide, methotrexate, chlorambucil, vincristine, vinblastine, mercaptopurine, and melphalan. Many people fear they will experience uncontrolled vomiting after receiving chemotherapy, but this side effect can almost always be controlled.

Tips for controlling nausea. Your doctor may recommend a number of medications that can control or lessen experiences of nausea. These antiemetic drugs are usually administered *before* chemotherapy actually begins so that the medication has time to take effect. Particular drugs and doses are sometimes changed until a proper fit is found to control your symptoms. Kytril and Zofran are among the newest and most effective antinausea medications.

Several classes of antiemetic or antinausea drugs help control nausea and vomiting. Antiemetics are often administered orally or intravenously, with their use continued through the period when nausea is expected to subside. *Phenothiazines* include Compazine, Trilafon, and Torecan. These are "old drugs" with moderate effectiveness against problems like nausea and vomiting. *Butyrophenones* include Haldol, Inapsine, and Innovar and are sometimes prescribed for nausea if phenothiazines don't work. *Corticosteroids* such as Decadron and methylprednisolone have antiemetic properties and are sometimes used with good results. *Sedatives or hypnotics* like Valium, Dalmane, and sometimes marijuana (THC) may be prescribed to reduce nausea.

Dietary tips for nausea. Prevention is a good strategy if the anticancer drug you are taking is likely to have a side effect of nausea. Don't force yourself to eat if you really don't feel like eating, or don't let family members try to force you to eat out of a mistaken sense of "trying to help." Avoid eating overly large meals during the times when you are likely to experience nausea. Rather than large meals, try sipping small amounts of soup, juice, or carbonated drinks that are neither too hot or too cold. Taking these liquids with a straw may help you avoid unsettling movement. Note that going on a fast before receiving chemotherapy will *not* prevent vomiting; fasting is not recommended because it interferes with good nutrition. Prevent dehydration during bouts of nausea by drinking small amounts of clear and cool beverages every fifteen minutes or so, and then gradually work your way back up to normal eating by taking small sips of water every several minutes. Increase the intake until you can tolerate a small meal.

Practical tips for nausea. You might try wearing loose-fitting clothes during and immediately after chemotherapy treatments. Try to avoid odors that bother you such as smoke or perfume, because for some people, odors trigger nausea. Loud noises and certain sights or images can trigger vomiting in some people, and in those cases it's recommended that you avoid what makes you sick. After eating, try sitting up in a chair rather than lying down. It may help you to avoid sudden changes in position that can cause something akin to motion sickness. Be prepared with buckets, towels, and washable linens in case of unexpected vomiting, which might occur someplace like in the car on the way home from a treatment, especially with a child. Keeping something like an airsickness bag on hand may increase your comfort level if you are afraid you will vomit at the wrong time. To control anticipatory nausea, you may benefit from some of the relaxation techniques found in chapter 16, such as deep breathing exercises. A bit of distraction, fresh air, and exercise can help many people stave off nausea.

Hair Loss

Alopecia or sudden hair loss happens to many people undergoing chemotherapy. Hair loss affects both men and women. It is the most visible side effect of chemotherapy, and although it is not physically painful at all, hair loss can be emotionally traumatic if it occurs. With some anticancer drugs, hair loss is almost a certainty, with others it's unpredictable. The actual extent of hair loss depends on the person and on the anticancer drug or drugs being taken. Facial hair, underarm, and pubic hair may be lost. Hair loss typically begins within three or four chemotherapy treatments; hair may fall out very gradually, in clumps, or even all at once. Stress and malnutrition can also cause hair loss. Fortunately, hair almost always grows back after the treatments are completed, and sometimes begins growing back even before then. Hair occasionally grows back thicker or thinner than before. Gray hair sometimes grows back in its original color. Ask your physician if hair loss is likely to occur with the treatment you are receiving, because it's a side effect you can plan for in advance.

Practical tips for dealing with hair loss. Having your hair cut short makes it appear thicker, and will help you minimize any problems you might have if you do lose hair. To minimize or slow hair loss, pamper your hair. Washing or shampooing hair will not cause hair loss in itself, but be sure to use a soft hair brush and a wide-toothed comb. Also use mild shampoo (preferably one indicated for use on damaged hair) and conditioner for fine or limp hair. Pat hair dry with a towel, or use the lowest settings on electric hair dryers when drying your hair, holding the dryer at least four inches from your head.

Do not have your hair dyed, and don't get a permanent during chemotherapy treatment. Do not use bobby pins, curlers, and don't put your hair in a ponytail even if you're a man. Wigs are available for both men and women. You may want to shop for a wig or hairpiece as a preventative measure, before you lose a lot of hair, because it's easier to match your natural color when you have hair to match. It may also be possible to borrow a wig—local offices of the American Cancer Society sometimes have "loan closet" programs that loan wigs to cancer patients who cannot afford to buy them. You may even need two wigs, if your treatment is expected to last a year or more. Real hair wigs can also be made from your natural hair, if you cut it off before it falls out, but these wigs are expensive. Other types of custom-made wigs cost as much as $3,000, and are made from fine natural hair, with a foundation of lace which is custom fitted to your scalp. Less expensive ready-to-wear wigs can be purchased for as little as $75. Ready-to-wear wigs use nylon foundations and usually a more coarse grade of hair, sometimes synthetic hair, but they come in a wide range of styles and colors right off the shelf. Take a snippet of your hair and a snapshot of yourself before hair loss occurs. You may want to be fitted for a wig, or select scarves, hats, or turbans to wear in case you lose your hair. During regrowth, continue to pamper your hair. Minimize brushing and hair styling. Use as little as possible of mousse, styling gel, spritz, and hair sprays. Avoid permanents or hair dyes until the hair is at least three inches long and scalp is no longer sensitive.

Other methods of dealing with hair loss. Two medical methods are sometimes employed in an effort to minimize hair loss, but neither works all the time. Both methods involve wrapping the head in an attempt to minimize the amount of chemotherapy drugs which can reach the hair follicles of your head. One method uses an ice pack to cover the scalp. The other method uses a sort of scalp tourniquet or blood pressure cuff, which is inflated at the scalp to a level that exceeds the patient's normal blood pressure. Both are applied before chemotherapy treatments are begun, and continued for several minutes after each cycle of chemotherapy is completed. These methods may be comfortably used for short-duration chemotherapy, but not for chemotherapy that lasts a long time. Sometimes these techniques don't work to reduce hair loss. Some oncologists avoid both methods, because they fear the sanctuary that is created near the scalp may provide a site for a metastasis of cancer.

Loss of Appetite

Anorexia or loss of appetite is fairly common for people fighting cancer, due to physical as well as emotional stresses. Beware of protein or carbohydrate malnutrition. Taste alterations in many foods can also occur due to chemotherapy's effects; the taste alterations that occur are different in every individual but can affect appetite. Some anticancer agents dry the lining of your mouth, which can make it difficult to eat or swallow. Antinausea drugs can also cause the problem of dry mouth, which usually disappears when you stop taking the medication.

Practical tips on loss of appetite. It is important to keep your body as fit and well nourished as possible through chemotherapy, and then afterward, to help prevent a recurrence of cancer. A good moderate exercise such as walking may help you work up an appetite. Some of the stress-reducing exercises in chapter 16 may help, particularly if your spirits are down, and a mild depression is repressing your appetite. Take heart in knowing that if your chemotherapy treatment is successful, and you achieve a complete or partial remission, your appetite *will* return as will your enjoyment of certain foods. Remember that cycles of rest are built into chemotherapy treatment, specifically to allow you to increase your intake of such essential nutrients as calories, vitamins, and minerals. Some tips for making your mealtimes more pleasant and nutritious are included in chapter 12.

Dietary tips if food tastes different. Eliminate the foods that bother you from your diet, and look for substitutes. Try substituting chicken or fish for red meat, if the taste of meat annoys you. Try roasted peanuts rather than salted peanuts, if salted peanuts taste unpleasant. Try a different method of preparation—microwaving rather than frying, for instance. Experiment. It is possible that you can find foods you might actually enjoy more than usual during chemotherapy. Experiment with different flavors and tastes. A zinc deficiency can accompany some cancer treatments, but may be remedied with a supplement containing zinc. Nutritional supplements such as Ensure pack a lot of calories into an easy-to-digest liquid form. A number of brands and flavors of these supplements are available, some milk-based and some non-milk-based, and you may want to experiment with these first to see if you like them, and then to determine if they help you retain your weight. Baby food is also quite easy to digest.

Dietary tips if you have dry mouth. Try drinking a bit more fluid than usual between and during meals, a total of eight or more glasses a day. Try a lip salve to keep your lips moistened. You might try lemonade or hot tea with lemon, which can stimulate your mouth to produce a bit more saliva. You may want to try eating softer foods, such as soups and puddings. Cold foods may be easier to swallow than hot foods. Simply sucking on lemon drops or sugar-free candy helps some people.

Fatigue

What physicians term bone marrow suppression is a common side effect of some chemotherapy drugs. Bone marrow suppression affects your body's ability to manufacture new red blood cells, and it can make you feel tired and fatigued almost all the time. A shortage of red blood cells means your body gets a bit less oxygen than normal, as one function of red blood cells is to carry oxygen from the lungs to all the parts of your body. This anemia can make you feel quite weak or fatigued. Other symptoms may include feeling dizzy, short of breath, or chilled. Pale skin and muscle weakness can be aspects of anemia. Dehydration, lack of sleep, and poor quality sleep are among the other factors that may contribute to fatigue.

Tips for combatting fatigue. Your doctor will do blood count tests frequently and may order a blood transfusion if red blood cell levels get too low. A prescription from your doctor could help you relax or sleep.

Practical tips for combatting fatigue. Get plenty of rest. If you can anticipate your periods of fatigue, plan ahead for them. Try to limit your activities to those you feel are essential. Ask someone to help you with the housework, or to drive you to the supermarket when you feel strong enough to shop. When getting up, get up slowly to minimize dizziness. Sometimes fatigue is a result of several factors, and some experimenting around may help you. Stress, worry, and anxiety are among the psychosocial factors that can be a significant cause of fatigue, and you might want to try some of the stress-relieving techniques in chapter 16.

Dietary tips for handling fatigue. Eat more foods rich in iron, such as liver, red meat, or green, leafy vegetables. For several hours before you go to bed, avoid foods containing caffeine such as coffee, chocolate, or colas. Meals may be organized in advance, with portions of dishes or casseroles frozen in smaller portions, so that the physical act of preparing and serving a meal doesn't exhaust your energies. Drink more water and other liquids to prevent dehydration.

Infections

Bone marrow suppression also affects the production of white blood cells, which are an important component of your body's immune system. White blood cells fight off most of the germs you normally encounter in the course of your life. Chills, fever, sweating, diarrhea, or redness or swelling around a sore or pimple may be signs of infection. Another sign is if you bruise easily.

Tips for treating infections. Your doctor can prescribe antibiotics to combat infections, so be sure to notify your doctor promptly if you see symptoms of infection appear. Don't take aspirin or any other medication to alleviate symptoms until you speak with your physician or nurse.

Practical tips to avoid infections. Fourteen days after treatment, the white blood cell levels usually fall to their lowest point, so this is when the possibility for infection is highest. Be unusually careful and clean during the time you are most vulnerable to infections. It is just common sense to steer clear of people who have infectious diseases such as measles or the flu. Minimize your exposure to crowds. Wash your hands frequently, before and after you eat or use the bathroom. Wear protective clothing or gloves when gardening or picking up after dogs or cats. Clean any cuts or nicks in the skin immediately, using soap and warm water followed by an antiseptic. Use an electric razor rather than a blade to shave your face or legs, and a soft toothbrush dipped in warm water to brush your teeth. Gently pat your skin dry after a warm bath or shower, and carefully clean yourself after each bowel movement. If you have access to a bidet, its use can make the act of going to the bathroom a bit more sanitary and help you keep yourself clean. Portable bidets which fit inside a regular toilet are available, too.

Dietary tips to avoid infection. Be careful to avoid uncooked fruits or vegetables, raw eggs, raw milk, and food items that may have been handled by others, as well as stagnant water.

A note about bladder infections. Bladder infections and other urinary tract problems can occur with chemotherapy, particularly if you experience nausea and vomiting or some other symptom that prevents urination, which is your body's way to clear the bladder and kidneys of chemical waste products. To prevent bladder infections, drink adequate amounts of fluids. Urinary tract infections have symptoms including frequent or urgent urination, burning sensation, off-colored or bloody urine, fever, chills and fatigue, or low back or flank pain. Your doctor may prescribe antibiotics or offer other suggestions to relieve these symptoms.

Blood Clotting Problems

Bone marrow suppression also affects the body's ability to manu-facture the platelets that help blood clot. You may bleed or bruise more easily than normal while undergoing chemotherapy. You may see small red spots under the skin or have unusual looking urine or stools. Your gums or nose may bleed. Once this type of bleeding has begun, patients must frequently go to the hospital for blood transfusions to replace red blood cells and platelets lost from bleeding.

Tips for blood clotting problems. Report any unusual symp-toms of this nature to your physician. Ask exactly what symptoms you might expect and what precautions he or she suggests. Always talk to your doctor before using medication, even aspirin or Alka-Seltzer, because some of these over-the-counter medica-tions thin the blood and slow down its ability to clot.

Practical tips to avoid blood clotting problems. Avoid poten-tial injuries. Be very careful not to injure yourself by not playing contact sports such as football or soccer. Avoid cutting yourself with sharp knives or kitchen tools. If you cook, wear a padded glove while handling hot dishes, and be careful not to burn your-self by avoiding very hot household objects such as heater vents and lit light bulbs. Wear protective clothing while gardening, and gloves while handling thorny plants such as rose bushes or cacti. Use an extra soft toothbrush dipped in warm water to brush your teeth. Blow your nose very gently, without applying pressure to your nostrils to minimize nosebleed.

Mouth and Throat Sores/Infections

Mouth and throat problems. Sores in the mouth or *stomatitis* may open you up to the possibility of infection from germs that live in the mouth. The tissues of the mouth and throat may be-come irritated, bleed, or become unusually dry. You may have trouble swallowing. You may have problems with cold sores, med-ically known as *herpes simplex*. Some people also get a yeast infection called *thrush,* which looks like little white patches on your gums or inside your cheeks. Inflammation or mouth pain can greatly inhibit normal eating or drinking.

Tips for mouth and throat problems. Mouth sores usually last only three to eight days, although they may affect your appetite for longer than that. Prevention takes time and attention, but it's much easier than medical treatment. Your doctor can prescribe an antifungal medication to control thrush. Many yeast infections respond to lozenges or throat drops that contain clotrimazole, or mouth rinses containing Mycostatin. Acyclovir, an antibiotic, can be prescribed to prevent the recurrence of *herpes simplex.* Kaopectate, milk of magnesia, or other liquid drugs are sometimes recommended to mitigate pain because they coat the sores and keep away the saliva. A combination of drugs may be necessary to achieve control in the most severe cases. If time permits, you should see a dentist or a periodontist before beginning chemotherapy. Always tell your dentist you are beginning or undergoing chemotherapy, and ask if he or she has any additional suggestions for keeping your mouth and gums clean.

Practical tips for mouth and throat problems. Generally speaking, keeping your mouth as clean as possible helps. Mouth rinses such as those using baking soda or those recommended by your doctor can help neutralize the acidic residue in your mouth. Commercial mouthwashes that contain salt or alcohol will irritate the soft lining of your mouth. Carefully use dental floss. It may help keep your mouth clean to carefully brush your teeth or dentures after every meal with a very soft toothbrush, using baking soda and water, or a nonabrasive toothpaste. Clean and then store your toothbrush in a dry place after use.

Dietary tips for mouth and throat problems. If your mouth or throat is sore, you may wish to eat cool, smooth foods like milkshakes, cottage cheese, or puréed vegetables and meats. Avoid spicy or hot foods that make your mouth sting. Liquid nutritional supplements such as Ensure and Sustacal are available at pharmacies and can be a good source of calories and proteins for some people at this time because they are not irritating to the mouth. Milk-free supplements are available if lactose intolerance is a problem. A diet containing adequate vitamins, minerals, and protein can speed the healing of mucous membranes.

Diarrhea

Chemotherapy can produce loose bowels or diarrhea because the cells in the intestinal tract are vulnerable to the effects of anti-cancer drugs and the body's natural response is to try to quickly rid itself of damaged cells. Diarrhea dehydrates the body and may block elimination of waste products through the urine if it continues for long periods of time, because of the body's natural tendency to conserve limited water. Diarrhea is sometimes accompanied by vomiting. Emotional stress, lactose intolerance, chemotherapy, or radiation treatment directed to the abdominal region, fecal impactions, and other factors including the use of antibiotics and sensitivities to certain foods can cause diarrhea. Along with losing water, you can also lose important minerals your body needs, such as potassium. Diarrhea may occur a week or so after a chemotherapy treatment.

Tips for combatting diarrhea. Always contact your doctor if diarrhea continues for more than twenty-four hours. If you have pain or cramping simultaneously, your doctor should be notified immediately. Some medications your doctor may prescribe include Kaopectate, Lomotil, Imodium, Omodiu, paregoric, cholestyramine, Donnatal, or Robinul. You doctor may wish to prescribe medication to relieve the diarrhea; although if you have an infection, he or she may want to prescribe antibiotics first. Consult your doctor if diarrhea continues after you have taken medication to stop it. Your physician may suggest that you go on a clear liquid diet for a day or two to rest your bowels, knowing that you can make up the calories you miss later.

Dietary tips for combatting diarrhea. Your fluid intake is quite important, so don't stop drinking. Try small amounts of water, fruit juice, soup, or even drinks such as Gatorade, a product formulated for athletes to replace lost electrolytes. The so-called BRAT diet of bananas, rice, applesauce, and weak herb tea can be easily digested and is used by many hospitals to control diarrhea. Avoid foods that may aggravate your bowels—milk products, raw fruits and vegetables, spicy, greasy foods, or even coffee and tea.

Constipation

Some anticancer drugs and some painkilling drugs can cause constipation, as can inactivity or poor diet. For example, some drugs used in chemotherapy such as vincristine and vinblastine, and other symptom management drugs such as narcotics and tranquilizers, can slow down the normal movement of the bowels. Emotional stress can be a factor, as can a lack of normal eating or drinking because of nausea or fatigue.

Tips for handling constipation. Your doctor can prescribe laxatives and stool softeners, some of which are as natural as olive oil or mineral oil. Only take laxatives under your doctor's supervision. You should *not* self-medicate for constipation by taking laxatives or suppositories before checking with your doctor. Enemas or suppositories have a risk of causing infection at the times when your blood count is low. Your doctor may prescribe a medication to stimulate the bowels. If your white blood cell count is lower than 1,800, you should avoid raw fruits and vegetables, including lettuce, which would normally be recommended as dietary remedies for constipation.

Practical tips for constipation. Regular and moderate exercise helps many people relieve this problem.

Dietary tips for constipation. Unless your blood counts are low or your doctor forbids it, try a high-fiber diet, including whole grains, fruits, vegetables, dried fruits, and fruit juices such as prune juice. Ideally, you should start the high-fiber diet *before* beginning chemotherapy treatments that might cause constipation. If you increase the amount of high-fiber foods you eat, you should also probably increase the amount of fluid you drink because the fluid helps the fiber work. Drink eight to ten glasses of fluid a day to avoid dehydration, and try more nutritional fluids such as juice, milkshakes, and eggnog rather than water if you feel the increased amounts of fluids are decreasing your normal appetite. Avoid refined foods such as white bread and candy. Also avoid chocolates, cheeses, and eggs, which can cause constipation.

Nerve and Muscle Effects

Some chemotherapy drugs, in some people, produce side effects that affect the nervous system or the muscles. The hands or feet tingle, feel numb, weak, or even burn. You may experience a loss of balance and have trouble with motor coordination. Sometimes the muscles can feel tired or weak or sore. Pain in the jaw or stomach and hearing loss can also be symptoms.

Tips on nerve and muscle effects. Use common sense when getting around. If you don't feel right, be careful. If your balance is a bit off, use handrails and supports wherever possible, or have them installed in the home. Ask for help if you need it. Report these types of problems to your physician.

Skin and Nails

Chemotherapy may result in minor skin problems such as rashes, redness, acne, itching, peeling, even a "dry look" or dry-feeling skin. *Pruritus* is an intense itching of the skin, which can be caused by dehydration or by some drugs used in chemotherapy. Some chemotherapy drugs or radiation therapy treatments may actually cause the skin to change in appearance, and occasionally to darken in color. Most chemotherapy makes the skin unusually sensitive to the effects of the sun. Since fingernails are just hardened skin cells, a related effect is that fingernails may become more brittle than usual, or change in color or appearance.

Medical tips for skin and nail changes. Let your doctor know if you develop a sudden or severe bout of itching, if you break out in a rash, or if you begin wheezing or have trouble breathing—

these can be symptoms of an allergic reaction. Ask about ointments or medications that relieve rashes and similar symptoms.

Practical tips on protecting skin and nails. Protect and pamper your skin and nails to prevent skin problems. Wear loose-fitting clothes. Wear protective gloves or clothing while performing chores. Take showers or sponge baths rather than long baths. Use creams or lotions when your skin is moist after a bath. Use water-based moisturizers. Keeping your face clean with medicated creams or soaps can help acne. Over-the-counter fingernail hardeners can help brittle nails, but discontinue their use if irritation results. Always protect your skin from wind and temperature extremes and from bright sunlight. Studiously drinking eight to ten glasses of fluid a day may help, too. It may help you to avoid unusually strenuous exercise. Cornstarch, baking soda, oatmeal, or soybean powder added to bath water can, in some cases, provide relief. Cool wet packs may help relieve itching. Train yourself not to scratch where your skin itches, because that irritates the skin and makes it itch even more. Stress-relieving techniques in chapter 16 may also be of assistance, because there may be an emotional component to this side effect.

Kidney and Bladder Problems

Some drugs used in chemotherapy can cause temporary or permanent damage to the kidneys or irritate the bladder. A few anti-cancer drugs cause the urine to turn orange, red, or yellow or to smell medicinal. Men may also experience a change in the appearance or color of semen.

Tips for kidney and bladder problems. Check with your doctor to see if the types of drugs you are taking can affect these organs, and ask what symptoms might be normal to expect. Always report unusual symptoms to your doctor. Some signs you should be sure to report include painful or frequent urination, discolored urine, and chills and fever.

Dietary tips for kidney and bladder problems. Drinking plenty of water and other mild fluids helps assure a good flow of urine through the kidneys and speeds the irritants out of your system as quickly as possible.

Puffiness (Fluid Retention)

Some drugs used in chemotherapy, particularly the hormones such as prednisone, may cause your body to retain fluid. Fluid retention will increase your weight even if you don't eat extra food. You may appear puffy in your face or other parts of your body. This side effect should be distinguished from a medical condition called *lymphedema*, caused by the backing up of lymph fluid in certain areas of the body after radiation therapy or surgical removal of lymph nodes.

Tips for fluid retention. Your doctor may be able to prescribe medicine to help your body shake off some of the excess water. Lymphedema occurs rarely, in either the chronic or acute form— to prevent it, work with your physician and a physical therapist to develop an effective exercise program and a good nutritional program high in protein.

Dietary tips for fluid retention. Avoid the excessive use of table salt, or foods with high levels of sodium such as TV dinners.

Tooth Decay

Some chemotherapy drugs will cause you to be unusually vulnerable to tooth decay and gum or periodontal infections.

Tips for preventing tooth decay. As previously mentioned, it's a good idea to see your dentist or periodontist before you begin chemotherapy. Have your teeth cleaned. Have cavities filled, dentures well fitted, abscesses, and gum disease treated if possible. Ask your dentist the best ways to brush and floss your teeth while you are receiving chemotherapy treatments. Your dentist may suggest a fluoride rinse or a gel to use each day that will help prevent unnecessary tooth decay. You may want to carefully brush your teeth after eating, using a very soft toothbrush dipped in warm water to soften the bristles before each brushing.

Sexual and Reproductive Problems

A person's sexual urges and desires, and even the sexual organs themselves, may be affected by chemotherapy. Your age, general health, and the type and length of chemotherapy are factors that affect the severity of side effects in this area. Men may experience infertility, lowered sperm counts, and other reactions. Women may find their ability to produce some hormones reduced, or sustain damage to the ovaries, resulting in irregular or halted menstrual periods. Women can experience a "false menopause," with symptoms such as hot flashes, itching, and discomfort or dryness of the vagina that can make intercourse painful and leave them vulnerable to vaginal infections. Men or women may experience a change of attitude about sexual intercourse as a result of either physical or psychological factors. Painkilling narcotics can inhibit sexual desire. In addition, experiencing some of the other physical side effects of chemotherapy will affect normal sexual function and desire, which may be either diminished or different in form during chemotherapy. For instance, pain makes it difficult to relax, but painkilling medications may lessen interest in sexual activities even as they relieve the pain. Emotional stress and powerful emotions such as anger, anxiety, and depression also greatly affect sexual desire in most people—and powerful emotions may be felt not only by the person receiving chemotherapy, but by the spouse or lover as well.

Tips for handling sexual problems. Most people need love and loving relationships more than ever during chemotherapy. Unfortunately, they may have a hard time accepting affection because they don't feel "lovable" because of changes in their appearance or attitude. For instance, women who have experienced a mastectomy may not feel that they are lovable without a breast, and dealing with this loss of body image will take patience and reassurance on the part of her partner. Men treated for prostate cancer may experience impotence. Prostheses such as artificial breasts and penile implants are available and will help make you comfortable as you move back toward normalizing sexual relationships.

Many people may find sexual issues difficult to discuss, and some changes in perception and attitude may be necessary to maintain a healthy sexual relationship. Oftentimes, professional counseling can be quite helpful.

Most people can live without sex more easily than they can live without love. Some individuals may wish to be touched and held more frequently, rather than just having intercourse. A partner may wish to change the time of day or the position used for sex. A vaginal lubricant may help women prepare for sex. Even though it may be difficult to begin discussing these issues, talk about your situation as fully as you can with your partner, who should also be made to understand that emotional stress may come along with your treatment and temporarily affect your own desire. Tell your partner that you still feel love for him or her.

Delivering love and affection may require huge adjustments on the part of both partners. Problems that were latent in the relationship may get worse. Couples who have been sexually active before chemotherapy very frequently find ways to continue sexual activity. Touching, sensual massage, and kissing are all sensual romantic pleasures, and they can be real and creative expressions of love. Gestures such as giving the other person little cards or presents can be important, too.

Give everyone time to adjust. Expressions of affection don't *have* to be physical. Note that many sexual problems have their roots in emotional issues rather than physical issues. Unfortunately, one partner may withdraw, leaving the other partner feeling abandoned. Rebuilding a relationship isn't easy. It might help either partner, or both partners, or the family to participate in a support group, in counseling sessions, or even to seek the services of a reputable sex counselor if adjustments are difficult.

Tips on handling reproductive problems. Prior to chemotherapy, men might want to deposit some sperm in a sperm bank as a precaution. This is most important to young men who have not begun families. Sperm banks are not to be found in every town, but are located in most large cities. A cost is involved in sperm banking, and a sample of sperm should be analyzed in a laboratory before deposit to assure a level adequate for fertilization. Men undergoing chemotherapy should plan to use effective birth control methods during intercourse, because anticancer agents can cause damage to chromosomes in sperm, and children conceived during chemotherapy may suffer genetic damage.

Unlike sperm banking, storage of eggs for women is not yet perfected. Egg storage is not recommended yet, because it is only done in research facilities. Nonetheless, women should seek to avoid becoming pregnant during chemotherapy, due to the possibility of birth defects in children conceived while undergoing chemotherapy. Upon the advice of a gynecologist, women already pregnant may want to delay the start of chemotherapy for a period of time until the fetus is developed enough to withstand its effects.

Women with vaginal dryness or itching may wish to change their style of dress to include loose, comfortable clothing. Using a water-based vaginal lubricant such as K-Y Jelly will protect against infection or injury to the mucous membranes during sexual intercourse. Any vaginal infection should be treated promptly. Women should watch for unusual discharges, and tell their doctor when their menustration usually occurs.

Reporting Side Effects

Your doctor will probably advise you which side effects might be expected with your chemotherapy and which should be reported, including the side effects that should be reported immediately. In addition to the side effects already discussed, some of the side effects to watch out for include fever, shaking, chills, bleeding, bruising, increased pain, uncontrolled pain, and any new side effects never experienced before including rashes, headaches, shortness of breath, and swelling.

Some side effects occur very rarely, but might be a cause for concern if they appear. As a general rule, while undergoing chemotherapy, anything you don't expect or understand relating to your body should be reported as soon as possible to your doctor or your cancer nurse.

Even when your doctor or nurse has warned you that you might expect a particular side effect, notify your doctor if the experience is worse than predicted, lasts longer than predicted, or makes you extremely uncomfortable. When in doubt, tell your medical team and let your doctor decide whether or not the symptoms you're experiencing are important enough to be treated.

Managing any side effects you experience will keep you sailing through chemotherapy treatment, holding fast to your aim to recover your good health. But physical side effects are only a part of the total picture. Good nutrition—dealt with in the next chapter of this book—is also of paramount importance to your recovery as are the other issues addressed in Part II.

OTHER ASPECTS OF CHEMOTHERAPY

---

*Great emergencies and crises show us how much greater
our vital resources are than we had supposed.*
WILLIAM JAMES

12

GOOD NUTRITION AND GOOD HEALTH

WHAT YOU EAT CAN HELP YOU HEAL

CHEMOTHERAPY AFFECTS THE ENTIRE GASTROINTESTINAL TRACT, BUT those effects may sometimes be mitigated. This chapter discusses the basics of good nutrition as it relates to cancer therapy and suggests ways to eat well and as nutritiously as possible during chemotherapy. Fortunately, you have some control over your eating habits. What you eat will help you keep up your strength and heal. As you will see, evidence suggests that a few of the major types of cancer may often be prevented by attention to diet.

This chapter contains information on maintaining your strength through good nutrition before, during, and after chemotherapy. Because chemotherapy often depletes your physical strength, you may experience some problems eating enough or eating well. Treatment can even cause malnutrition. Included here are suggestions to help you eat despite the limits your chemotherapy treatment may impose.

More Nutrients

Doctors estimate that people being treated for cancer have a need for 20 percent more nutrients than they would normally use.

There are several reasons why this is true. The physical shocks of surgery, radiation, or chemotherapy treatment can take a great toll on the body, causing it to burn enormous amounts of energy. For another thing, cancer cells can be growing quickly and vacuuming up a lot of nutrients such as vitamins, minerals, and protein from the bloodstream. Some evidence suggests that cancer cells actually release chemicals into the bloodstream that can either accelerate the consumption of nutrients, or suppress appetite. Psychological stress, financial worries, lack of sleep, and many other factors can cause the body to burn calories faster than normal. Remember, too, that the life span for each cell in the intestine is about two weeks. There may be periods when your appetite is low because chemotherapy treatments have temporarily knocked back the normal populations of these intestinal cells.

It is a myth that everyone loses weight during chemotherapy. Some people use food to comfort them during times of stress, and these people can actually gain weight during chemotherapy, particularly if their treatment involves the somewhat milder forms of adjuvant chemotherapy. Doctors do sometimes use protein and vitamin supplements as a medical treatment to restore immune system factors, but the extent of weight loss depends on the types of anticancer drugs administered, and an individual's response to chemotherapy. Depression and emotional worries can also inhibit your desire to eat because your state of mind is a factor, too, as are the attitudes you have about food and eating.

Psychological Comfort

The simple acts of eating and drinking have an important psychological dimension for many people, since they are relatively safe and sensual pleasures. Just finishing a snack or a meal normally leaves us with a comfortable, satisfied feeling.

If you're in a hospital, you may be stuck with hospital food unless you can afford to have all your meals catered, or find a sympathetic friend or relative who will bring you meals. As an outpatient, you have more control over what you eat. Your ability to nourish yourself during chemotherapy can hasten your recovery—or hinder it. Nourish yourself.

If you experience problems eating, you may have to just be patient with yourself, and ask others to do the same. Eat in a way that takes into account your physical limitations.

When you're having chemotherapy, some days you may feel like eating a lot, and other days you may not feel hungry at all. It is helpful to realize that many dieticians advise people being treated for cancer to keep within five or ten pounds of their normal weight. Staying within these guidelines allows you some room to add or drop a few pounds as your appetite fluctuates. If you wish to monitor your weight, you can check your weight on a bathroom scale at intervals, perhaps once or twice every day. If you don't have a scale, you can borrow or buy one.

Your doctor will be concerned if you lose an inordinate amount of weight. As a rule of thumb, a 5 percent weight loss will cause your physician some concern, while a 10 percent loss in weight should be seen as a clear danger signal.

Unfortunately, your eating habits can become an obsession for people taking care of you. Family members may innocently prepare you big, spicy, aromatic meals that you cannot possibly eat, don't like to smell, and don't even want to see spread out on a table before you. You may need to speak to these well-meaning people about your preferences and offer suggestions on how they might make your meals more pleasant and appetizing to you. A good place to begin looking for recipes to use and information on specific diets is the free publication *Eating Hints: Recipes and Tips for Better Nutrition during Cancer Treatment,* available free from the National Cancer Institute, whose toll-free number is listed in the Other Resources appendix of this book.

Nutritional Help

You may wish to find an expert on nutrition to guide you during this time in your life, even before you start chemotherapy treatments. Starting a program of good nutrition early can help you build your strength for what lies ahead. It is possible to design a diet that mitigates some of the effects of the chemotherapy drugs or other medications you may have to take. Eating nutritiously helps you retain as much strength as possible during treatment.

Chemotherapy depletes the body of a great many necessary nutrients, according to one certified clinical nutritionist. For instance, chemotherapy can deplete amino acids such as lysine, which nourish the mitochondria in the intestinal tract. The liver is heavily stressed because its normal job of filtering waste materials from the blood is greatly increased, since the liver also must remove the biological waste materials produced by chemotherapy. The antioxidant vitamins such as A, C, and E are often depleted by chemotherapy drugs as are minerals such as selenium and zinc, needed for protein synthesis especially in the immune system.

Nutritionists can help design a nutritional program that will help you maximize your strength under the stress of chemotherapy.

Harriet's Story

Before she began her second course of chemotherapy nine years ago, a woman we shall call Harriet, a public relations specialist, thought it prudent to visit a nutritionist to help her build up her strength for her newest battle against cancer. Harriet had defeated breast cancer several years earlier with treatment, which included chemotherapy, and this effort gave her some idea of what she might expect.

Prior to beginning chemotherapy, Harriet visited a nutritionist every two weeks, where she received blood tests and was given vitamin supplements according to tests of her red and white blood cells. Among other dietary changes, Harriet modified her intake of red meat.

"I looked at visiting a specialist in nutrition as a way of keeping myself stronger through the chemotherapy, and then as a way to build myself back up after chemotherapy treatments were over,"

Harriet says, noting that she continues to take the supplements and carefully watch her diet, simply as preventative measures. "I look at nutrition sort of like life insurance. I feel if I can keep my strength up using diet and exercise, maybe I won't have to deal with cancer a third time."

Some medical doctors specialize in nutrition, and they are often members of the American Society for Clinical Nutrition. Other qualified nutritionists might be members of the Society for Nutrition Education or the American Institute of Nutrition. Registered dietitians have an undergraduate degree and are certified by the American Dietetic Association.

However, do beware of "nutritionists" without professional associations, or with mail order degrees, since do-it-yourself practitioners are found in this field. While diet is a significant risk factor for cancer, and good nutrition may help prevent cancer, also remember that it is almost *never* possible to cure cancer through dietary changes or through vitamin supplements alone.

Lactose Intolerance

Even if you've never had a problem with dairy products, some chemotherapy drugs or radiation therapy may make you lactose intolerant, a condition in which your body is unable to process the milk sugar called lactase. If you have a lactose intolerance, dairy products will give you diarrhea.

If you suddenly become lactose intolerant, you should realize that most people return to normal after chemotherapy. For the time of your chemotherapy treatments, avoid eating milk and cheese products, except perhaps for acidophilus milk and cheddar cheese. Nonfat active culture yogurt and regular buttermilk can be tolerated by some people because the lactase is changed in these products. Soy milk may be substituted for milk in cooking, although soy milk has a chalky flavor and you may not want to drink it. Eating a bit of active culture yogurt a few times a day may help counteract diarrhea, if the diarrhea comes from antibiotics.

Drink Liquids

Chemotherapy patients are often advised to drink more liquids than they usually consume. This is to help the chemotherapy medication do its job against the cancer, and also to protect the bladder and kidneys. Drinking more fluid will help you quickly eliminate the chemical by-products generated by chemotherapy. For example, drugs such as cyclophosphamide can cause a condition called cystitis. Patients receiving cyclophosphamide are sometimes advised to drink as much as three quarts of liquid per day.

Cisplatin, dacarbazine, daunorubicin, doxorubicin, lomustine, methotrexate, mitomycin, and plicamycin are chemotherapy drugs that can actually damage the kidneys, so drinking lots of fluids is also recommended with these drugs. Most of the time, it doesn't matter what kind of water you drink. But note that a microscopic organism called Cryptosporidium is sometimes found in municipal water supplies in states such as Florida, so health authorities in those areas recommend that people with AIDS and people undergoing chemotherapy drink purified bottled water.

Help with Meals

Loss of appetite can be a real problem for people on chemotherapy. At this time in your life, you may be burning more calories than usual because of the emotional stress and worry of having cancer.

If you are the primary person who cooks and prepares the food, and you are also the person taking chemotherapy treatments, you may need to ask for some help. If you are married, perhaps your spouse could take over a little bit of the meal preparation, or hire or persuade another person to help you. You may be able to ask a relative or a friend to help out some of the time. Children may be asked to handle the tasks they can manage.

Many communities have a Meals on Wheels type of program, which may be available to bring food to your home. Call and inquire about such programs in your community. Meals on Wheels can be useful if you are single or live alone, or even to give your regular cook a break.

Some churches and religious organizations have volunteer groups that assist their church members by preparing food or helping with other tasks. Your physician, cancer nurse, social worker, or groups such as the American Cancer Society may be able to help you contact local programs.

Mealtime Tips

Here are a few ideas that may help stimulate your desire to eat and alleviate some of the hassles surrounding meal planning:

- *Plan meals ahead.* Making a shopping list planning each meal in advance may help, even if you don't normally plan your meals that way. If you feel better in the morning, do more of your work in the morning. Big dishes such as casseroles can be divided and frozen, then taken out later and prepared. If possible, divide tasks into several parts, which you can do one step at a time or parcel out to others. You might even want to make a shopping list and let someone else shop for you, or find a grocery store which will deliver to your home. You could pick out one part of the meal that you really enjoy doing, and leave the rest to other people if that is possible.

- *Jazz up mealtime.* Make your meals more of a festive event by changing your normal routine, by eating in a different location, by adding color to the plate, or even eating by candlelight with some nice music playing.

- *Make some meals social.* When possible, eat with friends or family members rather than eating alone. Don't hesitate to accept gifts of food from friends or family members, and be sure to tell them what you like to eat. Give people your favorite recipes and see what happens.

- *Create new dishes.* Think about trying new foods and recipes.

- *Avoid foods you dislike.* Stay away from your food favorites if you don't particularly feel like eating them. Try something else. If the smell of warm food bothers you, try eating the food when it's cold.

- *Exercise moderately.* Take a walk before meals, if that perks up your appetite. If you had a favorite noncontact sport, take it back up a little bit at a time as you feel ready.
- *Eat smaller meals.* Instead of three big square meals a day, eat small meals or snacks whenever you wish. You can sometimes snack on fluids instead of solid food, including high-calorie fluids such as milk and milkshakes if you can tolerate dairy products, or sweet fruit nectars and juices.
- *Think healthy.* Work into your diet as many foods you know are nutritious as possible, such as fruits and vegetables.

It goes without saying that your lack of appetite can also have psychological causes. If you feel depressed, worried, or anxious, channeling some of your time and energy into the stress-relieving techniques listed in chapter 16 might help bring back your appetite.

Common Sense

Within the nutritional community, people hold a variety of opinions about nutrition during treatment for cancer.

A more middle-of-the-road dietician might advise people undergoing chemotherapy to eat a high-protein or high-calorie diet because people may not feel like eating the quantity of food they would normally consume. This kind of diet provides more calories with less bulk than a normal meal and may be easier to eat if your appetite is depressed. If you need to increase protein consumption, they might advise you to eat more beans, nuts, peanut butter, eggs, cheese, even meat and fish that can be added to other cooked dishes. Powdered milk may be added to regular milk, milkshakes, and casseroles to increase protein. If you need to increase your calorie intake, you might be advised to eat a lot of things you would normally eat only in moderation such as butter or margarine, sauces, gravies, whipped cream, cream, and mayonnaise, as well as adding granola and dried fruits to dishes, and advised to sauté or fry foods rather than broiling them.

A more holistically oriented nutritionist would advise you to avoid highly processed foods, fats, sugars, junk foods with chemical additives, animal protein, and animal fat. This nutritionist might recommend you consume more high-fiber foods high in caratonoids, including lots of fresh fruits and vegetables, preferably organically grown. The more holistic nutritionist might recommend you increase your carbohydrate consumption from the fiber-rich complex carbohydrates such as whole grains, sprouts and seed sources. To this, the nutritionist might add vitamin or mineral supplements tailored to the person and the chemotherapy at somewhat higher levels (but not *dangerously* higher levels) than average daily requirements. Supplements might include amino acid supplements from something like rice protein, rather than soy or milk-based protein, which can cause allergic reactions.

Many doctors simply advise people undergoing chemotherapy to eat a normal, well-balanced diet. Consult a doctor, nutritionist or a registered dietician if you have questions about your diet.

Eating appropriately involves the use of common sense. Common sense tells you to stay away from high-fiber foods such as prunes if you have diarrhea, or from high-calorie diets full of sugars, salts, and starches if you are gaining weight. Your physician may also recommend a particular type of diet for you, based on your own circumstances and treatment, and you should work to follow your doctor's suggestions before you try anything else. Just to be on the safe side, ask his or her opinion about your other nutritional ideas. Most doctors go along with anything within reason, but they should warn you away from things such as megadoses of certain vitamins that have been proven dangerous.

If you drink, ask your physician about the use of alcoholic beverages. Alcohol can adversely interact with some drugs administered in chemotherapy and intensify normal side effects. In other cases, moderate amounts of alcohol such as a small glass or wine or beer before dinner may help you relax and increase your appetite a bit. Marijuana (THC) is legally available as an appetite stimulant, and works for some people, although it has its own side effects.

Exercise is good, but note that exercise affects people's desire for food in different ways. If exercise stimulates your appetite, you might want to exercise before dinner. If you don't feel like eating for a while after you exercise, you may want to hold off on the exercise until an hour or so after you eat. Do exercise as you can, even beginning in your hospital bed. Moderate exercise is an important part of a healthy lifestyle. Exercise has a number of wonderful benefits to overall health, in addition to its effect on appetite.

Cancer and Nutrition

Epidemiological or statistical studies have examined groups of people with predictable eating habits and turned up significant variations in incidences of certain cancers, which must be attributed to diet. For instance, Seventh-Day Adventists in the United States eat a strict lacto-vegetarian diet, and they have very low rates of colon cancer. Dairy product–loving Sweden has the world's highest incidence of ovarian cancer with twenty-one cases per 100,000 women, while countries that have much less fat in their diet such as India, Africa, and Japan have only three to four cases of ovarian cancer per 100,000 women. As many studies suggest, diet has a role in both bringing on and preventing cancer. The best conventional thinking is that 30 to 35 percent of cancers may have diet as a risk factor. On the high end, some doctors of nutritional science estimate that up to 70 percent of cancers may be related to diet.

Good nutrition is important before, during, and after chemotherapy treatment. There's no scientific evidence that dietary changes or vitamin supplements can stop a cancer from growing in the human body, but there's proof that good nutrition helps the body heal faster. Studies suggest that nutrition might often prevent the return of some types of cancer. Excesses and deficiencies in diet, particularly diets that are high in fat or low in fiber, are strongly believed to contribute to occurrences of cancer. Obesity is another recognized risk factor.

Daniel W. Nixon, M.D., author of *The Cancer Recovery Eating Plan,* divides cancers brought on by diet into cancers of what he calls "overnutrition" and cancers of "undernutrition."

Breast cancer, colon cancer, prostate cancer, pancreatic cancer, endometrial cancer, and even lung cancer have been linked to diets very rich in fats, what Dr. Nixon calls overnutrition. Generally speaking, people living in industrialized Western countries such as the United States whose diets are high in nutritionally complex meat and dairy products, and low in fiber, have a much higher incidence of these types of cancers than do people in the underdeveloped countries of the world.

Conversely, squamous cancers on the linings or coverings of organs, in the upper digestive tracts such as mouth, throat, and esophagus, cancer of the cervix, and stomach cancer are what Dr. Nixon calls cancers of undernutrition. These cancers occur more frequently in poor, underdeveloped countries where diets are high in fiber but often lack particular adequate vitamins, minerals, or other nutrients.

Some cancers have absolutely no known link to diet.

Preventing Cancer

Of all the many biochemical elements found in foods, the National Cancer Institute has identified more than one thousand substances that have some chemopreventative effects, at least in the laboratory. That so many substances in food have the potential of preventing cancer is itself an argument for eating a balanced diet, particularly one that includes unprocessed fruits and vegetables. It is also an argument against trying to get all your nutrients through vitamin and mineral supplements, which are chemically different than real food.

If you follow the American Cancer Society's guidelines listed below, you will probably get adequate vitamins and minerals in the foods you eat as well as a generally low-fat, high-fiber diet that will help prevent cancer. The American Cancer Society now recommends the following seven general guidelines to reduce the risk of cancer in all people:

1. Maintain a desirable body weight.
2. Eat a varied diet.
3. Include a variety of both vegetables and fruits in the daily diet.

4. Eat more high-fiber foods, such as whole-grain cereals, legumes, vegetables, and fruits.
5. Cut down on total fat intake.
6. Limit consumption of alcoholic beverages, if you drink at all.
7. Limit consumption of salt-cured, smoked, and nitrite-preserved foods.

Vitamins

Studies have begun to look at the effects of vitamins A, C, and E on various types of cancers, but these vitamins are not yet an accepted component of basic cancer therapy because their effects have not been proven. It is now medically accepted that people receiving chemotherapy with methotrexate for some types of tumors take a form of folic acid to decrease the toxic side effects. Promyelocytic leukemia is being treated with all-trans-retinoic acid, a form of vitamin A, with some improvements in some cases already seen. People with lung cancer have generally lower levels of vitamin A than most people, although it has not been proven that increasing any form of vitamin A will slow the development of lung cancer.

Vitamins A, C, and E have a role in cancer *prevention* because they are antioxidants that have an ability to clean up free roaming molecules known as free radicals, molecules believed to be crucial for the creation of cancer. Adequate levels of calcium and other minerals are believed to have a role in preventing some cancers, such as colon cancer. Zinc has an established role in healing.

Since people fighting cancer do need more nutrients, multivitamin and mineral supplements at moderate levels are recommended by some physicians, or at least not discouraged, but vitamins are *not* a cure for cancer in themselves. Many doctors and nutritionists warn against taking huge megavitamin treatments for cancer since many vitamins known to be good for you in moderate amounts can cause side effects if taken in excess.

For instance, the most prestigious advocate of megavitamin

treatments for cancer is Linus Pauling, a Nobel prize–winning sci-
entist who feels that large doses of vitamin C may help cancer patients heal faster after surgery or radiation therapy. But in *Cancer
and Vitamin C* Pauling writes that he is not so certain that large
doses of vitamin C are beneficial for people undergoing chemotherapy treatments, because the immune system can be weakened by chemotherapy and in some cases, megadoses of vitamin
C might actually help cancer cells reproduce.

Breast and Colon Cancer

The links to diet are clear between two of the most common cancers—breast and colon cancer.

Evidence of a link between dietary fat and breast cancer is
strong. Japanese women have much lower rates of breast cancer
than American women, a difference generally attributed to the
American high-fat diet and the Japanese low-fat diet. When Japanese women migrate to the United States and eat a more typical
American diet, their incidence of breast cancer rises. In animal
studies, too, increases in dietary fat are involved in producing
breast cancer and in helping it metastasize. Also in animal studies, a high-fat diet makes breast cancers grow, while a low-fat diet
suppresses the growth of breast cancer.

To prevent cancer in postmenopausal women completing adjuvant chemotherapy, or women on adjuvant therapy who are
gaining weight, Dr. Nixon recommends decreasing fat consumption to no more than 20 percent of daily calories, and increasing
fiber intake to twenty-five grams or more per day. Fruits and
vegetables which contain beta carotene, a natural precursor to vitamin A, may be particularly good to add to the diet as a preventative to breast cancer since these foods are also high in fiber.
Among the many foods containing beta carotene are apricots,
broccoli, and cantaloupe.

A high-fat, low-fiber diet is strongly associated with colon cancer. Adequate nutrition along with a low-fat, high-fiber diet is rec-

ommended. The evidence currently available suggests you can help prevent colon cancer from recurring with a diet containing adequate calcium, fruits and vegetables containing beta carotene, and foods such as garlic or onions from the allium family.

A low-fat, high-fiber diet such as recommended by the American Cancer Society is a very safe bet, particularly when combined with a healthy overall lifestyle, which includes moderate exercise, social encounters with friends and family, and no smoking. Several national health organizations now recommend that you eat 30 percent *or less* of your daily calories in the form of fat to reduce the risk of cancer, but some nutritionists such as Dr. Nixon believe that fat intake should be lowered to 20 percent for people who are at high risk for cancer. As a point of reference, the average American eats from 37 to 40 percent of their calories in the form of fat, much of this from animal products.

Lowering your fat consumption involves monitoring what you eat, and substituting some vegetables, fruit, and whole-grain foods for meat and dairy products. Having two or three meatless days every week is beneficial. The U.S. Department of Agriculture's food pyramid, pictured here, may also be helpful in meal planning.

When you begin to cut down your fat intake, it may be a shock the first time you look down at the highly recommended three-ounce serving of steak, which is about the size of a man's wallet. Add more vegetables and fruits to your meal, and that little steak soon won't seem so tiny after all. Even on a low-fat diet, you can get plenty to eat.

Among many other physiological benefits, good nutrition can strengthen your immune system. The vital importance of the immune system in maintaining health has been dramatically highlighted by the current epidemic of AIDS, which is associated with big increases in AIDS-related cancers such as Kaposi's sarcoma and non-Hodgkin's lymphoma. Practicing good nutrition will not cure these cancers, but good nutrition and a healthy lifestyle can *help* keep your body strong, so that your own immune system can do a maximum good job of both fighting disease and preventing recurrences.

FOOD GUIDE PYRAMID
A GUIDE TO DAILY FOOD CHOICES

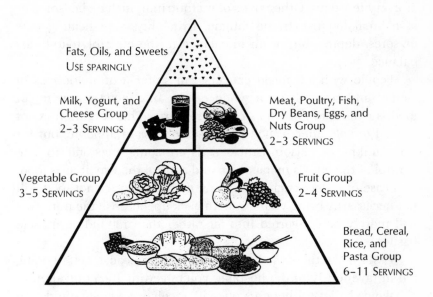

Fats, Oils, and Sweets
USE SPARINGLY

Milk, Yogurt, and
Cheese Group
2–3 SERVINGS

Meat, Poultry, Fish,
Dry Beans, Eggs, and
Nuts Group
2–3 SERVINGS

Vegetable Group
3–5 SERVINGS

Fruit Group
2–4 SERVINGS

Bread, Cereal,
Rice, and
Pasta Group
6–11 SERVINGS

Use the USDA's Food Guide Pyramid to help you eat better every day. Start with plenty of breads, cereals, rice, and pasta; vegetables; and fruits. Add two to three servings from the milk group and two to three servings from the meat group.

Each of these food groups provides some, but not all, of the nutrients you need. No one food group is more important than another — for good health you need them all. Go easy on fats, oils, and sweets, the foods in the small tip of the pyramid.

Malnutrition

Another risk is that inadequate nutrition or malnutrition can limit the amount of chemotherapy your body can tolerate, thereby decreasing the chances for successful treatment. There is a cycle in which a reduced appetite and weight loss feeds into fatigue and depression, which diminishes the appetite and creates even more weight loss. Clearly, in some cases, good nutritional management can literally save your life.

Loss of weight is the biggest single indicator of malnutrition, but it may be difficult to notice if you look at yourself every day and the weight loss is gradual. If you're an outpatient, monitor your own weight or have someone record it at set intervals, such as every few days. Other signs of malnutrition include bedsores or skin breakdown, extreme fatigue, irritability, slow-healing cuts or sores, depression, or an imbalance in the electrolyte-to-fluids balance.

People with advanced cancers can suffer a dramatic loss of weight and strength even when eating an adequate amount of food, a condition known as *cancer cachexia.* This condition is not related to side effects such as nausea or loss of appetite, but for some unknown reason, cancer cells are sometimes able to take control of the body's metabolism and control the way it uses food. In a case of cancer cachexia, eating more food or richer food will not necessarily bring your strength back up, because the nutrients will merely be converted into fat rather than rebuilding muscle tissues.

Don't make the mistake of thinking that because you're being fed intravenously in the hospital, you're getting the equivalent of a balanced diet, although you will receive adequate fluids. In some studies done a few years ago, between 30 to 40 percent of hospital patients were found to be malnourished.

If nutritional therapy is begun in the hospital, try to maintain it after you return home. Make sure you understand what kind of diet you should be following when you leave the hospital. Get as much specific information as you can. At some point, you may consider seeking the help of a good nutritionist or dietician to help you plan your diet and your meals. Good books and pamphlets are also available on this topic, and you can educate and help yourself. Remember that it's much, much easier to maintain good nutrition than to fight your way back from a condition of malnutrition.

If you're visiting the hospital as an outpatient, you'll have much more control over what and when you eat. Use your freedom to keep yourself as strong as possible during chemotherapy and beyond. If your healthy diet allows you to have a bit more energy, you may be more up for maintaining your physical appearance, the topic of the next chapter.

13

YOUR APPEARANCE

LOOKING GOOD MAKES YOU FEEL BETTER ABOUT YOURSELF

THIS CHAPTER CONTAINS TIPS FOR KEEPING UP YOUR PHYSICAL appearance, since chemotherapy treatments may affect your appearance in a number of subtle ways and indirectly affect your self-image and self-esteem. Loss of hair is an obvious concern to many chemotherapy patients, but changes in complexion and sensitivity to sunlight are other side effects that affect your personal appearance.

For many people, going back to work or even going to the supermarket for the first time after chemotherapy treatment can be traumatic. Just looking in the mirror tells you that your body has undergone some changes, and these changes will be quite visible to you even though other people may not even notice them. You may feel quite self-conscious for a while.

But you can learn ways to manage the temporary changes to your appearance that chemotherapy may bring. Fixing yourself up will give your ego a lift. Improving your appearance may even make you feel more social, and make you a bit more fun to be around. If you need a prosthesis, get one. When you're more comfortable about the way you look, you may feel more capable of handling the slings and arrows of the outside world.

The American Cancer Society's "Look Good, Feel Better" program is one major effort in this direction, and it is popular not only among women, but also with children and men. These free programs are offered in many communities, often in concert with local cosmetologists who have experience or special training in dealing with cancer patients. Many major cancer hospitals also offer personal image programs as part of a multidisciplinary approach to treating the whole person. Exercise, nutritional, and stress-relieving programs may also affect the way you look, making your face and your body appear more relaxed because you actually *are* more relaxed.

Experimenting with changes in your appearance, with different colors and looks, and taking sensible precautions to protect your skin may help you keep up your appearance while undergoing chemotherapy treatment.

Changing Your Appearance

Fear of changes in appearance such as the loss of hair or loss of weight, and stress when change occurs, is as normal as happiness and joy when the fallen hair or the lost pounds begin to return. If you're worried about your appearance, think about what might help you deal with this stress. If you lose or gain a little weight, you might want to buy yourself some new clothes. Worried about losing your hair? According to one cosmetologist, one straight-laced mother had her hair cut in a mohawk a few days before she expected to lose her hair, an offbeat but empowering move for her, which made her children scream—but gave her a kick. Many women like to have a wig matched to their normal hair before they begin chemotherapy treatments, but some just go *au naturel* with their bald heads and make a sort of fashion statement. Hats, turbans, and scarves can create a nice look. Men can also begin wearing a hat or get a toupee if they are concerned about their looks.

Experiment with Colors

If chemotherapy changes your complexion, and it frequently does, you may find you look better in bright colors rather than beige, peach, and yellow, which may make you look even more washed-out. Men or women may experiment a little with brightly colored scarves, shirts, sweaters, tops, and ties. If you are a woman, your customary makeup may need to be modified to make you look your best. Experiment with different colors of makeup. Even if you don't wish to change the colors you wear, you may feel more comfortable during chemotherapy if you modify your style of dressing, since loose-fitting garments are often more comfortable. With children, particularly young girls, the steps to take depend a lot on how the child's peer group accepts her appearance.

Protect Your Skin

Chemotherapy often makes your skin very sensitive, so you'll have to take care to protect it—your body's largest organ. To protect your skin from the sun's damaging rays, many doctors advise that you wear sunblock of no less than 15, PABA-free, preferably a block that is water-resistant or waterproof. Apply sunscreen *before* you go outdoors. Plan to apply sunblock to your entire body, even the parts covered by clothing, which can also burn. Use lip balms in addition to suncreen, too. Note that blotches on the skin can result from overexposure to the sun during chemotherapy, and although the blotches will go away, you'll look better if you don't get them in the first place. One hundred percent ultraviolet protection sunglasses are also recommended, because you can get cancer in your eyes if they are overexposed to sunlight. Don't forget that your skin is fragile and will be much more sensitive to sun than normal. Wear a brimmed cap even in the early morning hours when sun exposure is not normally a problem. The Skin Cancer Foundation advises people with all skin types to avoid direct sunlight from 10:00 A.M. to 3:00 P.M. Sunlight is even more intense at locations such as the beach, lakes, or in snow.

Even people who normally have oily skin may have problems with dehydration during chemotherapy. Doctors may recommend an over-the-counter moisturizing lotion you may use. Women should use alcohol-free toners and avoid astringent-type products, which may cause premature wrinkles. Women's foundation make-up should have a sunscreen added for additional protection from the sun's rays.

To prevent the infections that may enter your body through your skin at times when you are vulnerable to infection, it's a good idea to keep little alcohol prep pads in your purse or pocket to make sure the things you touch in public places are clean. For women, for instance, wiping off eyebrow pencils and lipsticks you may try at a department store cosmetics counter assures that the objects you come in contact with are superclean. Men may want to wipe off exercise or office equipment. Any item that might carry germs can be wiped clean and sanitary with these little pads.

Other steps to avoid and prevent infections may be taken during chemotherapy. Among other dangers, a fungal infection can occur under artificial fingernails, moving from under the nail directly into the blood, and this infection can be fatal if your immune system is quite depressed. So don't wear artificial fingernails when undergoing chemotherapy. Your scalp, too, may be quite sensitive whether you've lost hair or not, so don't dye your hair or get a permanent during or immediately after chemotherapy, because these procedures may irritate your sensitive skin. If you take precautions to avoid infections, you can go out into the world without a great deal of worry—to shop, to visit, or to work. Just getting out may lift your spirits a bit, and that may help your appearance.

Appearances Are Important

Your appearance may change, but experimenting a bit with colors, clothing, and dress styles may be quite helpful in maintaining your physical appearance—and your spirits—during chemotherapy. Inside your body, where no one else can see, chemotherapy can also disrupt your life. Many people with cancer experience some physical pain, the topic of the next chapter, but any serious pain you experience can be relieved.

14

PAIN

THIS COMMON SYMPTOM
CAN BE CONTROLLED

PAIN IS ONE OF THE MOST COMMON SYMPTOMS EXPERIENCED during cancer and cancer treatment, and it's also one of the most subjective. Pain is either *acute,* or sharp and sudden, or *chronic,* and just always there. Just because you're being treated for cancer doesn't mean you have to endure physical pain, which is frequently a combination of both physical and emotional factors.

Medical researchers estimate that 30 to 45 percent of patients being treated for cancer experience moderate to severe pain at the time of diagnosis and intermediate stages. An estimated 75 percent of patients with advanced cancer experience pain. Doctors participating in a recent National Cancer Institute workshop on cancer pain declared, "The undertreatment of pain and other symptoms of cancer is a serious and neglected public health problem."

Prolonged pain can decimate your overall quality of life, and it increases the stress on caregivers because they will be frustrated if they cannot help relieve your suffering. Pain control is increasingly being seen as a *right* even among terminally ill patients such as those with AIDS, where pain management techniques are quite similar to those used for patients with cancer.

While undergoing chemotherapy, you do not have to be like the stoic heroes of old Western movies, who bit a leather strap when a doctor yanked the bullet out with a pair of pliers, because in those days, heroes had no choice but to endure pain. Today, many methods of relieving pain are available to you. Your doctor has many pain-relieving drugs and medications, which can soothe even severe pain. You can also experiment with nonmedical methods to relieve your own pain that have worked for other people, an empowering tactic that may give you a double benefit by relieving pain and improving your quality of life.

Causes of Pain

Pain has many causes. Pain during cancer treatment can result from many factors including nerve damage from the growth of a tumor, invasive procedures such as operations, toxicities from chemotherapy or radiation, infection, or even aching muscles due to a lack of exercise.

The emotional meaning that some cancer patients attach to pain is great, because many wrongly take pain as a signal from their body that death is near. This connection is primitive and almost irrational. Psychologically, pain can be linked to anxiety and depression, which can exaggerate or amplify its effects.

Pain generally adds stress, slows healing, and debilitates your body. It can decimate your quality of life by diminishing your strength, sleep, appetite, concentration, sex life, family life, and even your appearance. Untreated and uncontrolled pain can increase your suffering on many levels, including the psychological, social, and even the spiritual level of your life. Prolonged pain can even lead some people to reject tenaciously held religious beliefs, or to flee from medical treatments, which can save their life.

The medical community is becoming more aware of the need for pain control. Pain has been found to be undertreated in both adults and children. In a statement published by the National Cancer Institute in 1990, a panel of physicians indicated that "every patient with cancer should have the expectation of pain control as an integral aspect of his/her care throughout the course of the disease."

Fortunately, pain can be managed effectively in more than 90 percent of cancer patients using relatively simple means.

Describe Your Pain

The first step in alleviating any pain is to describe it to a medical professional. Tell your doctor what you are experiencing, or have someone else tell him or her. This goes for chronic pains you experience, or all new or acute pains that cause you a problem. Communication is important in all your relationships during chemotherapy treatment, but perhaps most crucial, and sometimes most difficult, is communicating the particulars of a pain to a medical oncologist who may seem hurried and rushed. Get over the idea that your doctor "can't be bothered" with hearing about your aches and pains. Gather your courage and tell him or her about it, in a way that defines the pain accurately enough for the doctor to arrive at a course of action.

To describe pain accurately and clearly, tell your physician the following:

- Where pain is located
- When the pain began
- What type of pain it is (i.e., dull, sharp, or throbbing)
- Where it is located, and if and where it moves
- How often you have it
- The severity of the pain itself
- What you have noticed that relieves the pain, and what you have noticed that makes it worse
- Medications you've tried before and how they work
- Methods of pain relief that have worked for you in the past
- Any symptoms that accompany the pain, such as sweating or nausea

This information is important. If you find it difficult to speak out in your doctor's office, write this information down and take it with you. Tell your doctor about the pain, and ask for help. If you're using nonmedical techniques such as meditation or visual imaging that give you some relief, be sure to mention those. It is important to keep your physician abreast of what you are doing to manage pain, as well as any problems with pain that linger or remain.

Nonmedical Techniques

Nonmedical pain-control techniques do exist. The least invasive pain-control techniques won't necessarily involve your doctor. For instance, for some adults, sexual activity can relieve mild pain in some situations. Hypnosis and acupuncture relieve pain in others. Just having a parent present has been shown to help relieve some pain in children being treated for cancer, presumably because it calms the fears of the child.

Many stress-relieving techniques do truly relieve pain. Relieving pain certainly improves the quality of your life, and scientific evidence exists that pain relief can extend the average life span of groups of cancer patients, particularly if the patient has been taught techniques to employ to reduce stress or relieve pain.

When the strength of the evidence and its consistency are considered, three of the most effective pain-relieving techniques are hypnosis, relaxation therapy, and imagery. Interestingly, procedural information provided to patients and their families as to how their illness will be treated is also an effective technique to control pain. Other nonmedical techniques that work include distraction, exercise, acupuncture, transcutaneous electrical nerve skin stimulation (TENS), biofeedback, pastoral counseling, psychological counseling, and support groups. Even listening to music has a documented pain-relieving effect.

Instruction in many nonmedical pain-relieving techniques is now offered to patients recovering from cancer at comprehensive care cancer hospitals as part of the multidisciplinary approach to treatment. Techniques to relieve stress or pain are discussed in more detail in chapter 16, and you may want to experiment with some to see which work best for you.

The use of nonmedical pain-relieving techniques has several

benefits. For one thing, you may need to take less medicine to achieve pain relief. The techniques you use may also significantly affect your own attitudes and your own personal sensitivity to pain, since you are empowering yourself. Putting yourself on a program of pain or stress relief will give you a hand in your own treatment, and that will give you a feeling of control. It stands to reason that if you feel you're more in control of your own life, you won't be as vulnerable to obsessing about particular aches and pains.

Take note that while nonmedical techniques may relieve pain or stress in themselves, they are typically used to *supplement* medications prescribed by your doctor. But please don't hesitate to share results of techniques that work best for you with your medical treatment team, because other patients may also find them to be of value.

And even beyond these methods, don't forget that the pastimes and activities that relaxed you before you were diagnosed with cancer may still help distract you from your physical worries. You may still enjoy curling up in a favorite chair with a good novel, watching the college football games on Saturday afternoon, or sorting through stacks of old photographs to organize the family photo album.

Pain-Relieving Drugs

Medical oncologists can prescribe a wide selection of pain-relieving drugs called *analgesics* ranging from mild to potent, which help control pain.

Today, the least invasive drugs such as oral, transdermal and rectal medications are used to manage pain in more than three-fourths of all cases. More rarely used are stronger and more invasive techniques including intravenous and subcutaneous drugs and epidural and intrathecal analgesics. The most invasive techniques, including nerve blocks or palliative surgery, are used only on a few patients. In the most severe cases, these techniques can help patients whose pain has not responded to medications or other techniques.

Levels of Treatment

To assure a rational treatment of cancer pain all over the world, the World Health Organization has recommended that physicians utilize a "ladder" of analgesics or painkillers, and begin treatment using the mildest medications first. The first rung on this ladder are mild painkillers with few if any side effects such as aspirin or acetaminophen (Tylenol), typically administered as pills, which should be tried first for mild to moderate pain. For mild pain, two or three tablets is a typical dose. After these is a relatively new class of painkilling drugs called nonsteroidal, anti-inflammatory drugs (NSAIDs). The NSAID drugs include ibuprofen, diflunisal, and naproxen, which are slightly more effective than aspirin. The upset stomach experienced by most people who take these pain-relieving drugs can be alleviated by taking NSAIDs with antacids such as Tums, at mealtime, or in combination with another mild drug called sucralfate. The NSAID drugs may also be effectively used in combination with narcotic medications, allowing the use of fewer narcotics to control more severe pain. Antidepressant drugs such as amitriptyline, given at bedtime, can sometimes help control pain although some people can't tolerate the "spaced out" feeling this medication brings.

Narcotics

If these drugs do not relieve pain, doctors may administer the milder narcotic drugs such as codeine or Percodan. Reserved for the most severe pain are stronger narcotic drugs such as morphine, methadone, or Dilaudid.

Morphine is the standard against which the stronger narcotic drugs are measured, and it has been in medical use for many years. Morphine is a mood elevator, and it helps to lift the spirits of some patients, which is a benefit. When high enough doses are administered, morphine can relieve all but the most extreme levels of pain by heavily sedating the patient so that he or she literally feels no pain.

Forms of morphine such as Roxanol and MS-Contin are now available in pill form, which eliminates the need for injections while effectively controlling pain. These morphine pills are longer lasting morphine preparations that need to be taken only two or three times per day. Hydromorphone is available in many forms including as a rectal suppository, an advantage when the patient is vomiting and unable to keep a pill down. In this case, a suppository allows the pain-relieving narcotic to remain in the system.

For fleeting or temporary pain, doctors may prescribe combination drugs such as oxycodone plus acetaminophen, or codeine plus acetaminophen, on an as-needed basis for pain relief. When the pain is chronic, physicians may prescribe stronger narcotics such as methadone or morphine along with full-strength NSAIDs. Side effects of narcotic medications include constipation and nausea, and some people become agitated, confused, appear very sedated, or have difficulty breathing. These drugs also have a tendency to accumulate in the body.

Fears of Addiction

A persistent myth, which still pops up in patient-doctor conversations, is that the use of narcotics to control pain will result in drug addiction. Many patients fear becoming addicted to narcotics, and some doctors are leery of their use for the same reason. You should understand that if you are given narcotics to relieve pain, it is drug *dependence* that may result. Drug dependence is different from drug addiction, which has a strong psychological component. In the past, many doctors also feared addicting the patient and did not prescribe adequate doses of narcotics to control pain. Pain relief is a right. It is another myth that morphine is only given to patients who are expected to die.

Physicians and major cancer organizations such as the American Cancer Society are currently working to assure cancer patients that fears of drug addiction are overblown when it comes to pain control for cancer. If narcotics are used over an extended period of time to control pain, and the patient does become drug dependent, doses of the narcotic are gradually tapered off to avoid the agony of withdrawal symptoms once the crisis has passed.

Cancer patients, and particularly terminal cancer patients, have a right to be relieved of pain by whatever means are available. If the pain-relieving medication prescribed by your doctor isn't working, be sure and make that clear to your medical team.

Special pain clinics and pain management programs are beginning to appear in major hospitals around the country. For a listing of these facilities, contact the American Pain Society, listed in the Other Resources appendix of this book.

The first resort for pain control should be your medical team, although other stress-relieving techniques can help. You need to communicate the particulars of your pain to your physician, and assert your need for pain relief. Pain has both a physical and an emotional component, of course, and both are important. A discussion of the emotional issues involved in cancer treatment begins in the next chapter.

15

EMOTIONAL STRESS

How to Weather Your
Emotional Storm

CHEMOTHERAPY ENGAGES YOUR BODY, BUT TREATMENT FOR CANCER has an emotional and social impact that few people are able to ignore. In your own heart, you'll experience plenty of powerful feelings during chemotherapy. Unfortunately, you'll have to deal with this psychological and social turmoil simultaneously with the physical turmoil inside your body. Keeping a positive attitude about your treatment and working to communicate how you feel to those around you may provide some shelter from this emotional storm.

Emotional, social, and even spiritual stress may inhibit your immune system, drag down your spirits, and slow your recovery from cancer. Although a bit of stress adds pizzazz to life, too much mental or physical stress just drains the quality out of your life like water out of a bathtub. Fortunately, a lot of stress may be relieved.

In comprehensive cancer treatment hospitals, the multidisciplinary approach to cancer treatment involves a lot of participation from people who work in an area called "supportive care." Sometimes called complementary care or alternative care, supportive care basically aims to support your chemotherapy treatment with help in other areas of your life. Psychologists, chaplains, social workers, pharmacists, nutritionists, sex coun-selors, pain management specialists, and rehabilitation therapists are some of the professionals who may compose a comprehensive cancer hospital's supportive care team, which is typically headed by a physician. Visual imaging classes, hypnotherapy, patient ed-ucation, and support groups legitimately fall under the umbrella of supportive care, as do pet therapy, art therapy, music therapy, heat and cold therapy, a humor cart, skin stimulation, and acupuncture. The goal of supportive care is to enhance the qual-ity of your life during and after medical treatment when you're staying in a hospital, and many of these services are free.

If you're an outpatient, many of the stress-management tech-niques worked into hospital supportive care programs can be learned and applied on your own. You can help yourself. After all, you will support your medical team's efforts when you relieve your own emotional pain and stress, and that will increase your body's natural ability to heal.

Positive Attitudes

There is plenty of anecdotal evidence that patients with a positive attitude are more likely to recover from illness, and that what used to be called "the will to live" is extremely important even in this high-tech medical world.

Morris Abram, a prominent New York lawyer diagnosed with hopeless lymphocytic leukemia on his fifty-fourth birthday, beat cancer with an unusually aggressive course of chemotherapy. Reflecting on his experience, Abram wrote that his positive re-sponse to chemotherapy may have been helped along by his pos-itive attitude and his stubborn will to live.

"I resolved the night of the diagnosis that I would not yield; I would not die; I would seek the most aggressive help available and take any risks for the chance, however small, to live," he wrote in 1979. Abram suffered ferocious physical side effects during chemotherapy, but he also found the strength to try a few legal cases while he was being treated. "I don't think there's any ques-tion but that there's some kind of nexus, as yet undiscovered, between one's emotional well-being and perhaps the endocrine system," Abram believes.

A few years ago, a young engineer undergoing chemotherapy was visited in the hospital by his stepmother, a physician. She saw the young man flat on his back and marveled at his ferociously upbeat attitude and his apparent lack of fear. Despite the obvious effects of chemotherapy on his body, the young man was without a shred of self-pity. He was clearly focused on defeating the disease and getting on with his life—which he very shortly did.

"You just have an incredibly positive attitude," the young man's stepmother told him, admiringly patting his shoulder.

"I don't know how else to act," he replied.

Norman Cousins contributed the insight that laughter positively affects our bodies, whether it comes from the much-discussed placebo effect or not. The power of giving and receiving love is quite well known. Even smiling can punch up our immune systems, according to a research study done by Dr. Paul Ekman of the University of California at San Francisco.

"How can the cancer patient achieve hope?" asks Harold Benjamin in *From Victim to Victor.* "You can foster hope by meeting or becoming aware of ex-cancer patients—the more the merrier; by keeping up your social contacts; by paying attention to recovery statistics; by deriding myths and fables that surround cancer and recognizing that they don't apply to you; by becoming aware, at your most conscious level, that as long as statistics show that even if one person recovers from the type of cancer you have, there is every reason to hope you will be that one; and, finally, by 'acting as if' you have hope. So take all of these actions," Benjamin advises cancer patients.

Benjamin says that medical evidence is accumulating that positive emotions may prevent illness by offsetting the damage to the body caused by negative emotions such as anger and depression. But whether you call people who work to help themselves get well "patients active," as does Benjamin, or "exceptional patients," the term used by Bernie Siegel, any patient becomes active and exceptional when taking steps to display optimism, personal courage, and a stubborn will to live.

Role Changes

Nobody lives in a vacuum. Living through a bout of cancer may cause our lives to change dramatically. When our roles in life change, our perceptions of ourselves and others change, too.

If you think about it, your own self-image is tied up with any number of things in the world around you. You define yourself by your work, your interests, your economic status, your neighbors, your social life, or your family. When you're undergoing chemotherapy, it may not be enough to define yourself as an account executive, a caring grandparent, or a good neighbor. You may lose your sense that the old rules and roles still apply. You may find you are required to adjust great portions of your life to your physical condition, which involves dealing with a lot of painful perceptual changes at work, in your economic circumstances, and within your social life and family.

Dealing with changes at work. When people are ill, they can't do what they can when they're at the top of their game. Undergoing chemotherapy could mean making changes in your work habits, whether you're a corporate president or not. If you don't function as well as you did before treatment, this may cause a *lot* of anxiety for you and the people who work under, over, or around you. On the other hand, it doesn't *have* to be an issue at all. Recognize that changes in our abilities affect our feeling of accomplishment, and our feeling of being comfortable enough to let our hair down and relax with co-workers. People undergoing chemotherapy or recovering from cancer may fear the loss of their job or subtle attempts to ease them out of the company. For retired people, frustration may occur simply in the changes that illness brings to a leisurely lifestyle, or at the monkey wrench that chemotherapy tosses into a comfortable and predictable daily routine.

Dealing with changes in economic circumstances. It can be enormously expensive to be treated for cancer, whether health insurance is paying a portion of the costs or not. In addition, other costs such as transportation to and from the hospital, child care, and even the costs of wigs, prostheses, and more, which may not be covered at all under some health insurance policies. Worse, you may not even *have* health insurance. These days, the loss of one income in a two-income family can be downright traumatic. The financial aspects of being treated for cancer and some helpful suggestions may be found in chapter 18.

Dealing with changes in your social circles. The number of people in your social life may shrink for many reasons during your treatment for cancer. You may have to make efforts to keep parts of your social circle intact, or to expand it and make new friends, perhaps in a support group. If you're suffering from physical or mental fatigue, you may not feel like doing some of the things you normally do, such as attending a seminar or convention, actively participating in your church or synagogue, or playing in a bridge game or mixed bowling league. Some people within your social circle may avoid you because they believe that cancer is contagious. Others may stay away because they're making a misguided effort to help you keep your strength. It is discouraging when a friend or acquaintance stays away. You must make a conscious effort to communicate with people you know, and to not withdraw from your own life. You may also have to manage some things alone.

Dealing with changes within the family. If your chemotherapy treatment requires a stay in the hospital, treatment at home, or even time at home in bed to convalesce, family members may need to pitch in and help in new areas. Children may need to assume more of the household chores, for instance, or get a part-time job to help the family finances. A spouse unaccustomed to managing the family's finances may be forced to do so. Mowing the lawn, cooking Sunday dinner, or dressing a child for school are minor events in most people's lives, but they can seem like insurmountable problems when the person who normally does them is not well enough to perform those tasks.

Changes in family roles may have profound emotional complications. If you're the person responsible for something that doesn't get done, you may feel guilty and angry at yourself because you feel you're letting your family members down. And just when you want them to be quiet and be helpful, your children may need a lot more attention, reassurance, and even more discipline than usual. Take care of yourself first, but explain as simply as you can that you are trying to get well. Give your children what attention you can. You might ask a family member or friend to spend some extra time with them, or even to take your spouse out to see a movie. If you're an unusually proud or self-sufficient person, you may not find it easy to ask anyone for help or assistance for what seems like the first time in your life. Make the effort. If someone offers to help, give the person something useful to do.

Taking on more than you can physically or emotionally handle can be frustrating, stressful, and exhausting. If you're being cared for at home and you can't handle everything, simply rethink what you must do and establish priorities. Focus on what is truly most important at this moment. Let the minor tasks slide away, or delegate them to someone else. If the family structure can't handle all the additional demands, consider hiring professional nurses or housekeepers if you can afford them, even for a day or two a week. Perhaps a relative could be asked to help out on a temporary basis, to give the caregiver some time off. Some churches have volunteer groups that can be quite helpful. Hospice organizations can help with terminally ill patients. Unfortunately, even when you seek help, you may not find it every time. But you will feel better if you make the effort.

Changes in roles and duties can be more than uncomfortable. For instance, just standing quietly by the side of a family member or friend undergoing chemotherapy can be difficult, especially if the patient does not think to thank you, or acknowledge your sacrifice. Resentments need to be quickly brought out into the open and discussed honestly, instead of being covered up and allowed to smolder. Discussing painful issues isn't easy, and mentioning something one time may not completely resolve it. But resentments will build up faster if issues are continually glossed over, or if a tense situation is dragged out over a long period of time.

Emotional Stress

Note that you will not become mentally ill just because you are treated for cancer. However, your emotions may run riot as your mind wrestles with all the confusing new information and doubts about the future. Your psychological ups and downs may well be magnified under stress.

Before, during, or after chemotherapy, you will experience changes in your body, your mind, or in your life's routine. If you obsess over these things, and if you see them as permanent losses rather than changes, you'll begin to think they're overwhelming. The mere idea that you're going to start chemotherapy may make you feel like you're clutching the bar on the front cart of a roller coaster just beginning to head down the biggest, steepest hill in the world.

In addition to whatever physical side effects you may experience, your primitive "fight or flight" response to danger may be triggered continually as you confront the modern version of beasts in the jungle. You may experience psychosocial shocks during chemotherapy treatment and in other areas of your life, and your reaction to these threats will leave you emotionally exhausted.

Understand that the greatest amount of emotional stress hits most people at a few key points, including right after the diagnosis of cancer, upon beginning chemotherapy, after their chemotherapy treatment has been completed, or when they are released from the hospital. It is even normal to feel anxious when you return for physical checkups long after your cancer is in remission—and to feel relieved when your tests show everything is fine.

Feelings are elusive but quite powerful. Even if you are diagnosed with a small, easily cured cancer such as skin cancer, the first feeling you will experience is a stomach-curdling fear. Fear of death is a basic, primal emotion experienced by almost everyone who is told he or she has cancer. The frustration, fear, and confusion that attend a period of real or even anticipated physical helplessness may trigger outbursts of rage, or even knock you into a mind-numbing depression. At some point, you may angrily ask the unanswerable question, Why me?

Powerful feelings such as anger, fear, and depression can create emotional storms in almost any person, especially if the emotions are bottled up, and not directly dealt with or even acknowledged. Just admitting to yourself that you feel emotional stress is a first step. Try to identify what emotions you feel. Next, try to figure out exactly why you feel the way you do. Identify your emotions, sort them out, and try to figure out what triggers them.

"Anyone can become angry—that is easy. But to be angry with the right person, to the right degree, at the right time, for the right purpose, and in the right way—this is not easy," Aristotle wrote in *Nicomachean Ethics.*

If you're continually angry, for instance, try to figure out just exactly why you are angry. Talking this out with other people may help. Employing one or more of the stress-reduction techniques listed in the next chapter may help. Crying, or even screaming into a pillow, relieves stress in some people.

Taking positive action that will help and not harm you is the key to riding out your emotional storm. The emotional roller coaster ride that accompanies chemotherapy will get a little smoother if, like the woman in the following story, you can make plans to deal with stress in a positive way.

Janette's Story

A young woman we will call Janette, a teacher and a mother of two children, had several weeks to plan a stay in a comprehensive care cancer hospital after she was diagnosed with colon cancer. With her husband and friends, Janette sat around the dining room table and mapped out a strategy to make her hospital stay as pleasant as possible.

When she was admitted, Janette brought some items from home such as a colorful afghan, pillows, and some of her own house plants and flowers, which "took the cold edge out of the hospital room." A friend who composed music made a special tape for her. During her chemotherapy treatments, she listened to relaxation tapes from a psychologist as well as tapes of her favorite music on a small portable cassette player.

In the hospital, Janette received ninety-five-hour cycles of fluorouracil, at three week intervals, as part of her treatment, which included radiation therapy. "I knew that if I survived it I would be a better person. I was really enraptured to find out how many people were willing to go to such great lengths for me," Janette recalls.

"Friends were with me when the chemotherapy started each time, which helped a lot. Having a support system was really helpful," Janette says. "Once you're in a treatment program you feel better, whether it's chemotherapy or whatever. You feel better once you're engaged in a battle plan."

Janette used imagery and visualization and visualized her treatment as horses stamping cancer cells to bits. She kept two journals, one of which was medical and involved writing down the doctor's comments, and one which was very personal and upbeat. She sought the help of a psychiatrist to help her resolve the anxiety she felt, which included the fear that she would die and leave her children without a mother.

Her husband did not deal with the situation well, and he withdrew for a time. Her family hired a housekeeper to relieve the stress of housework and child care. When she was in the hospital, Janette visited with her young children in a beautiful formal garden at her hospital.

About a week after chemotherapy, Janette experienced side effects including heavy exhaustion and mental fatigue. She remembers vomiting for two days after the second treatment. Her skin turned black, she experienced thirty square inches of third degree burns, and sore and watery eyes.

But with a little help from her friends, Janette survived chemotherapy treatments. Her colon cancer is now in remission, and she has passed the period of greatest danger for recurrences of cancer. Janette now says the experience has given her a greater appreciation of life. She's gone back to doing some things she once loved, such as shoeing horses and competing in horse shows.

Fear

Understand that it's quite normal to fear what the American Cancer Society has identified as the "Five Ds"—death, disability, disfigurement, dependence, and disruption of important relationships. In one research study, about 40 percent of all cancer patients report having psychological problems that are associated with their disease. Thirty percent said they needed help managing their daily life or coping with pain. Between 15 to 20 percent reported problems with housing, neurological function, family support, finances, or nutrition. Fifteen percent said they were very concerned about their physical appearance. Another 7 percent had needs in communication or transportation. Some people reported problems in several areas.

Unfortunately, cancer treatment can be an emotional nightmare. Some of the powerful feelings you might experience include anger, fear, loneliness, anxiety, dread, resentment, helplessness, panic, sadness, irritability, depression, a sense of unreality or irrationality, and certainly a feeling that you've lost control over your own life. You may feel like a leaf in the wind, drifting about in the grip of huge faceless forces you cannot control. You may feel like the Italian poet Dante, who opened *The Divine Comedy* with the line, "In the middle of the journey of our life, I found myself in a dark wood, where the straight path was lost."

The shocks of medical treatment can be emotionally profound, and experiencing the power of your own feelings is quite another matter from reading or thinking about them. As an extreme example, the emotion of fear is so powerful that physicians have documented a few medical cases where patients see their diagnosis of cancer as a death sentence and literally "frighten themselves to death." These people so dreaded the idea of death by cancer that their fear actually caused their own death to come faster than it could have possibly occurred from cancer even if the cancer was never treated.

Realizing that you are experiencing emotional stress doesn't necessarily mean that you and your family should go right into counseling. It should be noted that psychological and social problems weigh heavily on the minds of many people being treated for cancer. However, counseling helps many people get through troubling periods in their life. If you think counseling might help, try it. Taking positive action to speed your own recovery will lift your spirits and allow you to improve the quality of your life.

"I felt so good when I walked out of the counselor's office. If I'd known I wouldn't be charged for it at the hospital, I might have gone in a long time before," laughed one good-natured woman now cured of cancer, who got a lot of benefit from her first trip to a professional counselor in the hospital.

You can help yourself get well. Despite the availability of more medical information than ever before in the history of mankind, people still have misconceptions about chemotherapy or cancer. Good information will help eliminate some fears. Working to eliminate fear in yourself and your family will help a lot, because fear is contagious.

Patients like Janette find that a bit of advance planning before chemotherapy treatments, or before going into the hospital, can make chemotherapy much easier on a practical level. If the obstacles you face seem completely overwhelming, remind yourself over and over again of the things you've already achieved in your life, including the difficulties you have faced and overcome. Remember your own displays of personal courage. This will help put the challenges you face in their proper perspective and help you reconnect with the strength that you've already exhibited in your life.

Communication

Talking about how you feel can help relieve some of the emotional stress associated with chemotherapy treatment. Even social contact with another person *without* mentioning your feelings may make you feel better. Several research studies have shown that people generally live longer lives when they are not isolated from other people.

Many cancer patients have admitted that open communication within their families is a significant problem. Unfortunately, not everyone in your life is going to know when you wish to discuss your feelings. Even sensitive, caring people frequently hold back, waiting for their cues from other people. Realize that the person being treated for cancer has the *responsibility* to indicate when he or she is ready to talk. Your friends and family members may be not talking to you because they are waiting for a signal from you. They may think they are protecting you by not discussing things they fear will upset you. Friends and family members may avoid even asking questions because they "don't want to bother you when you're sick."

Communication is a two-way street, and the street may be blocked at either end. Chemotherapy patients certainly have feelings they need to communicate. Relatives of cancer patients have needs, too, that need to be addressed. Make Today Count, a support group for cancer patients and their families, was begun by newspaperman Orville Kelly, who had an insight into all the bottled-up feelings cancer patients need to share when he returned home from one of his chemotherapy treatments and talked about how he felt with his family for the first time.

Good Communication

If you are receiving chemotherapy, communicate, communicate, communicate. Be sure to talk about good things, such as positive test results or a positive response to treatment. After you've talked about the positive things, it's all right to mention the things that really annoy and trouble you, too.

Whether you're a patient or the relative of a patient, what you should aim for is something in between the two dead ends of the communications spectrum—at one end the unrelieved depression of "woe is me," and at the other end the phony cheerfulness of "everything will always turn out fine." When you are able to strike an honest balance somewhere between these two extremes, you may help other people do the same.

Making an effort to create good honest communication within your family is a good place to start. Even if you are uncertain about the future, talking about your worries with the right people at the right time, in an honest, straightforward way, will help you come to terms with your uncertainties. As you've already learned, upset feelings are normal. Don't forget there are already strong feelings in the air, and that you're not the only person who has limits, or who has a need to talk.

If you're *not* ready to discuss the details of your illness with someone else, try to find a way to communicate that without hurting the other person's feelings if he or she happens to broach the subject. You might say, "I'm glad you're interested in my health, but I'm not ready to talk yet." When you are ready, give the people around you permission to discuss your treatment. You might begin by talking about how you feel, without pressuring the other person to say anything back immediately. When a misconception or a myth pops up in conversation, be ready to contradict it.

People typically indicate with verbal clues and body language that they wish to talk, since an estimated 80 percent of communication is nonverbal. Apparently idle conversations, spending more time than usual with family members, fidgeting or appearing nervous, or even just staring off into space may be signs that a certain family member wishes to talk to you, but doesn't quite know where or how to begin. Politely give that person a cue that it's okay to talk. When the other person speaks, listen to what he or she has to say.

Understanding exactly what worries you may be helpful in figuring out how to lessen its impacts, especially if the cause of your worry has a practical solution. If you fret that your three-year-old daughter might fall down the stairs, for instance, perhaps you can figure out a way to prevent her from getting to the top of the stairs. If you have temporarily lost your hair and feel embarrassed about it when you go out in public, perhaps you might buy or borrow an attractive wig or hat. If you worry that your wife and your children may someday wind up in an ugly legal battle over your estate, call a lawyer and make a will in which you clearly specify your wishes.

Make an effort not to withdraw from your children or your friends, your social life, or from doing what you are able to do around your home. When you are back home after a visit to the

POSITIVE THINKING

Sometimes positive thinking is just a matter of asking yourself the right questions, or turning negative thoughts on their head. Examples:

Wrong: What's the use of trying?
Right: What's the use of *not* trying?

Wrong: I can't forgive myself for having cancer.
Right: I *can* forgive myself for having cancer.

Wrong: My life is not worth living.
Right: My life *is* worth living.

hospital or doctor's office, simply staying in touch with the world around you and the things you normally do in your life can relieve stress. Going back to your usual work may be beneficial, when you can do that, because it may take your mind off your physical condition. Permit yourself some time to recuperate and to ease back into your life.

As you move through chemotherapy, you may find good days intermixing with bad days. Learn to savor the good days, and to appreciate life's fine, small moments. Tolerate the bad days as gracefully and courageously as you can, and do have patience with yourself and your own body. Permit yourself to express all your feelings, especially the pleasant ones such as joy, love, happiness, and laughter. "Be not afraid of life," wrote American philosopher William James in *The Will to Believe.* "Believe that life *is* worth living, and your belief will help create the fact."

Emotional stress is real, and changes in your life may well whip up a storm of strong feelings during your treatment for cancer. Remember that you can relieve a lot of stress by simply taking positive action to do so. It will help you to channel your strong emotions such as anger, fear, and depression into productive activity—including some of the stress-relieving techniques listed in the next chapter.

16

STRESS-RELIEVING TECHNIQUES

METHODS YOU CAN USE TO RELIEVE
PAIN AND EMOTIONAL DISTRESS

THIS CHAPTER INCLUDES A SURVEY OF NONMEDICAL TECHNIQUES that you may use to relieve emotional stress or pain. These techniques include hypnosis, imagery and visualization, biofeedback, rhythmic breathing, muscle relaxing techniques, distraction, and exercise. Some techniques must be learned in formal classes, but can be repeated on your own time in your own home. A few require the presence of an expert practitioner. Others require no formal training, just a bit of time. All these techniques help a lot of people—and may also work for you.

A Stanford University study of breast cancer patients published in 1989 showed that women who were taught self-hypnosis techniques for pain control and participated in a support group for breast cancer patients lived thirty-six months longer—*twice* as long as women in the control group who received the same medical care without the support services. In similar research at other institutions, positive results were achieved with patients who had lymphoma and lung cancer. One study of AIDS patients measured the immune system's response to support groups that focused on coping and relaxing skills and found that the immune systems of patients in the support group were actually stimulated, as shown by the "natural killer" (NK) white blood cell levels, which were higher in the patients in the support group.

In addition to giving you a sense of control over your own life, and focusing your energy to "fight back" against cancer, many of the stress-relieving techniques listed in this chapter will improve the quality of your daily life and make possible a more comfortable convalescence. Emotional, social, and even physical stress or pain may often be alleviated with the following coping and relaxing techniques. When you are comfortable or relaxed, your own efforts will be most focused and effective.

Remember that all the techniques listed here have given *many people* relief. They are not dangerous. In fact, it's very safe to experiment in this area. Your emotional load will lighten when you find a technique which works for you. If you want to attend classes that teach these techniques, your doctor, nurse, or social worker can refer you to an instructor in your area.

Stress-Reducing Techniques

Many techniques have been proven to reduce stress, including a few methods that have been in use for hundreds of years. Some of these include rhythmic breathing, meditation, yoga, hypnosis, imagery and visualization, and biofeedback.

Rhythmic Breathing

You can use the technique of rhythmic breathing almost anytime. Rhythmic breathing will relax you, and it can create a good state of mind for other stress-relieving exercises, or for medical situations you face. One way to do rhythmic breathing is to get in a comfortable position and look at any distant object. Breathe in and out through your nose, counting in your mind to assure you spend about the same amount of time breathing in that you do breathing out. Repeat this in cycles until you feel relaxed. Audiotapes that instruct you on relaxation techniques are available at many bookstores, drugstores, and health food stores.

Meditation or Yoga

If you really like the rhythmic breathing technique, or if you want to take the concept a bit farther, you could try taking some transcendental meditation classes where more advanced breathing and meditation techniques are taught, or yoga classes where breathing techniques are combined with stretching exercises.

Hypnosis, imagery and visualization, biofeedback, and some other stress-relieving techniques are best learned from a trained instructor, although once learned they may be used anywhere.

Hypnosis

A trained hypnotist can put you in a trancelike state that will reduce your tension or discomfort. After contracting polio when he was only seventeen, and almost dying, the famous psychiatrist Milton Erickson trained himself in a form of self-hypnosis so that he could learn to walk again. You can also be trained to hypnotize yourself to relieve your own anxieties before chemotherapy treatments, or you can practice self-hypnosis to help relieve physical pain when it occurs. The American Society of Clinical Hypnosis listed in the Other Resources appendix of this book can provide referrals to professionals trained in the clinical application of hypnosis.

Imagery and Visualization

Using the power of your own imagination, you can actually relieve stress by simply imagining that your body is being helped or healed. This mind-body technique was developed by a radiation oncologist, Dr. Carl O. Simonton, and his psychologist wife Stephanie Matthew-Simonton. The Simontons don't claim that their techniques take the place of medical care, but they are confident that imagery and visualization can be quite useful as a supplement to medical treatment. In 1981, they produced data that showed that using imagery and visualization increased patient survival time. "It is our central premise that an illness is not purely a physical problem but rather a problem of the whole person, that it includes not only body but mind and emotions," they wrote in their book, *Getting Well Again: A Step-by-Step Guide to Overcoming Cancer*.

Imagery and visualization techniques are typically introduced after you are familiar with and using other relaxation techniques such as rhythmic breathing. These techniques can be learned in five-and-a-half day treatment courses involving cancer patients and their spouses at the Simonton Cancer Center in Montecito, California, which lately has begun incorporating music therapy into their program. The Simonton Cancer Center will also provide referrals to medical professionals in your area who have been taught their techniques. Another source is to look in your local phone book under "hypnosis" and ask for a referral to a person who teaches meditation techniques, which are similar. Imagery and visualization may be looked at as a movie you're making to control cancer—produced by, directed by, and starring you.

One way to visualize your own healing is to imagine that a globe of bright healing energy is forming in your body, and then "move" it with your mind to any part of your body where you have pain, tension, or discomfort. Another way is to try "visualizing" your own body's battle against cancer. You can imagine that your chemotherapy is an army of knights in armor, or even a high-tech version of *Star Wars* blasting away the cancer cells. Or you can imagine your white blood cells gnawing away at the cancer cells as a part of your body's response to the disease, or visualize your chemotherapy as a flock of birds pecking cancer cells out of your body. Basically, you visualize a response to cancer that seems interesting and effective to you.

Biofeedback

Biofeedback involves simple machines that help make you aware of when your body is relaxed and when you are tense. Simply put, you receive feedback when your body relaxes. Using biofeedback techniques to make you aware of your stress levels, you will eventually be able to control your relaxation responses without the machines. The Association for Applied Psychophysiology and Biofeedback might refer you to a clinical person in this area. Closer to home, your medical team may be able to refer you to a reputable person trained in biofeedback.

Acupuncture, acupressure, art therapy, music therapy, pet therapy, skin stimulation, and even patient education classes have also been found useful in helping people deal with emotional stress or physical pain.

Other Techniques

Other techniques to reduce stress include muscle relaxation, distraction, and practically every form of exercise. You don't need special instruction in any of these stress-reducing techniques, although exercise classes are offered almost everywhere. You can do many of them at home, as needed.

Muscle-Relaxing Techniques

Lie down, get comfortable. Take a deep breath and tense a group of muscles such as the muscles in your shoulders as hard as you can for a second or two while holding your breath. Then exhale and relax your whole body as completely and thoroughly as you can. Take another deep breath and tense another group of muscles, and then relax it. Some people start at the toes and work their way up to the top of their heads in this manner, or vice versa. Tensing and relaxing your sets of muscles takes a few minutes, but afterward you should feel as relaxed as if you'd just taken a warm bath.

Distraction

Watching a soap opera, reading a book, fixing a leaky faucet, petting the dog—these are all examples of distraction. Anything that takes your mind off your medical condition is a distraction. Distraction can relieve stress and make the time pass faster if you find the experience pleasant or interesting. As Norman Cousins pointed out in *Anatomy of an Illness,* the simple act of laughing has a therapeutic emotional effect; laughter can relieve pain because its physical effects include the release of natural painkillers called endorphins.

The act of listening to music, singing, or playing a musical instrument has been shown to be therapeutic with direct effects on both body and spirit. You may experience music alone; in fact, sometimes it's more pleasant that way.

If you're more social, you may enjoy doing something you've thought about but put off in the past, such as volunteer work. This can be something as simple as making a telephone call to another person who needs to talk. Helping someone less fortunate than yourself will distract you from your own troubles, and allow you to participate in life in an active, positive way.

Exercise

Exercise has several well-known benefits, and not much downside if it's done in moderation. Walking is a wonderful exercise. And some research indicates that exercise may actually prevent cancer. A recent study of premenopausal women at the University of Southern California showed that women who worked out between one and three hours per week actually lowered their risk of breast cancer between 20 to 30 percent, while women who exercised four or more times a week had a 60 percent lower risk of breast cancer when compared with women who were not physically active. The women who exercised participated in team and individual sports, ran, walked, worked out in a gym, or participated in dance or exercise classes. Another study of Harvard men showed that men who exercised frequently had a lower incidence of prostate cancer than men who were sedentary.

According to breast cancer survivor Nancy Bruning, author of *Coping with Chemotherapy*, exercise helps rebuild strength you lose by lying around in bed during cancer treatment. Just three days of bed rest can decrease a person's stamina by 25 percent, Bruning says.

Bruning cites the following benefits of exercise during chemotherapy:

- *Your spirits rise.* It's not just the release of endorphins or natural painkillers into your bloodstream, although that's important. Exercise helps you accomplish something physical, to take control of your body, and to feel more vital, disciplined, and alive. Exercise can even put a little fun back into your life, which is always needed.
- *Your energy increases.* Your heart, lungs, and muscles get a workout and get stronger. Your endurance and stamina will naturally increase.
- *You may experience less nausea and/or vomiting during chemotherapy.* Bruning's own queasiness during treatments was quelled to a great extent by swimming, an exercise that she loved. Exercise diverts blood from the gastrointestinal tract and into the limbs and muscles, she noted, and muscles don't have the ability to get queasy.
- *You'll help strengthen your immune system.* White blood cells in particular are strengthened by exercise, according to some studies.

Exercise can result in better sleep, a sharper memory, and enhance good moods. Exercise is also an excellent tool for regulating weight, Bruning notes. If you're in danger of losing weight, exercise might help you improve your appetite. Conversely, if you are gaining weight, exercise might give you something to do other than eat—and help burn calories and keep the pounds off.

Exercising with another person may make the activity safer and more fun, particularly at first when you are getting your "sea legs." Start gradually, exercising lightly perhaps twice a day. Work your way up to more strenuous exercises. You may work with a personal trainer who will take into account your medical condition. You can even start exercising when you're in the hospital if you like, by asking your doctor or a physical therapist to give you exercises you can do when you're in bed. Exercise will help you strengthen your body. If a particular exercise feels too difficult, skip it and come back to it when you feel like it. As a precaution, check with your doctor about the limits you should place on any physical activity during or after chemotherapy.

The techniques included in this chapter aren't the only ones you can use, although they certainly can help you. Support groups, counseling, and better communication techniques may also help you deal with emotional stress. Sometimes, it takes a combination of time and effort to work through and adjust to all the upheavals in your life.

Applying some of the techniques you've learned in this chapter may well help you relax during some of the emotional turmoil you experience during chemotherapy. However, no person lives in a vacuum. Sometimes you may not have an idea where to turn for help—or even where to begin looking for emotional support. Where to find emotional support is the subject of the next chapter.

17

OTHER PEOPLE CAN HELP YOU

About Your Emotional Support Bank

YOU MAY FEEL LIKE THE LONELIEST PERSON IN THE WHOLE WORLD after you've been diagnosed with cancer, but if you'll look around you'll probably see that you have several potential sources of support. Social and emotional support can spring from not only medical personnel, but also family, friends, and individuals and professionals in other areas. The resources available to you within yourself and within other people are probably much greater than you might imagine.

Certainly you can discuss a lot of things with a lot of different people. Your own personal support network might include people from your medical team, including doctors and nurses, as well as counselors, social workers, family members, friends, co-workers, support groups, or even your experiences with a higher spiritual power. Look at this network as your emotional support bank.

Medical Team

You can confide your feelings to doctors or nurses, if you feel comfortable doing so. Some doctors can be quite compassionate, but others won't be comfortable discussing nonmedical issues.

Oncology nurses usually have more time to listen, and although many are good listeners, most of their training is in the practical realm. Doctors and nurses can be good sources of referrals to other sources of support.

Counselors

Clergymen and clergywomen, psychologists, psychiatrists, even sex therapists are some of the professionals who might help you cope with the changes in your life through counseling. You may find personal therapy or even group therapy helpful. Although support groups are different from group therapy, you may also benefit from participating in one whether you're staying in a hospital or not.

Psychologist Lawrence LeShahn says a good rule of thumb when deciding whether to use the services of a hospital psychologist is when you feel your anxieties are overcoming your own ability to think clearly and make good decisions. Depression, extreme confusion, or a lack of vision into the future may all be reasons to seek out the services of a psychologist, he adds, and it's quite possible that you might find a good one. The same criteria can be used even if you are not hospitalized. Group therapy, in which several people meet together to work through their different concerns with a trained counselor, is a more comfortable and less threatening setting for some people.

Even if you haven't been a regular at church or temple, don't be embarrassed if you feel a need to talk with your rabbi, clergyman, or priest. Simply call this person and tell them you wish to talk. They will not deny your request. If you're receiving treatment in the hospital, most hospitals have a chaplain to whom you can speak. You can request to speak to a chaplain even if you are being treated as an outpatient. Don't be ashamed to try any type of counseling. You may benefit. Reputable counselors are professionals who are trained to help people get through very difficult situations.

Social Workers

If you receive medical treatment through a hospital, social workers can be of great help in dealing with many of the problems you may encounter during chemotherapy treatment, such as how your illness impacts your family. Social workers can be fountains of practical information, and a resource for information about support groups or therapy for either you or your family members.

Dianne R. Morrison, a former social worker who is now director of Total Quality Management (TQM) Services at USC/Norris Comprehensive Cancer Center, tells the story of a mother who was having radiation therapy treatments for cancer. The woman's daughter was ostracized by the other kids on the playground. At first the mother speculated the girl's playmates might be afraid of "catching" cancer. But the social worker eventually determined that the girl's playmates thought her mother was "radioactive" and were avoiding the girl because they were afraid of being irradiated. Explaining to the girl how radiation therapy really worked was a first step in combatting the playground misinformation. Another step was getting the girl in a play group with children of well cancer patients, indirectly giving the girl helpful experience with which to deal with her mother's cancer treatment.

Social workers can help bridge gaps between established medical practice and individual patients in the area of discharge planning where they frequently work. Morrison recalls a particular male patient who was in the last stages of terminal cancer and scheduled to return home. Part of the hospital staff's preparation for the patient's home care was the shipment of a hospital bed to the patient's house where his wife was waiting for his return. The bed was sent and sent again, but the patient's wife refused to accept delivery of the hospital bed. When the social worker contacted the wife, the woman regaled the social worker with stories of the couple's previous marital beds, which the social worker soon realized were important personal symbols of their marriage. What was going on was that the woman could simply not tolerate the idea of her husband dying in a strange bed while he was in their family home. The social worker then broke precedent and canceled the order for the hospital bed, making special arrangements for the man to go home and be cared for in the family bed.

If you are not receiving chemotherapy in a big cancer center hospital, you may ask your oncologist or cancer nurse to direct you toward a local source of social support. The American Cancer Society should be able to put you in touch with sources for emotional and practical help in your community.

Within Your Family

The renowned physician Harvey Cushing once noted, "The task of the physician is to protect the patient from the patient's relatives so that nature can heal him."

There is more than a grain of truth in Dr. Cushing's wry observation. Family members shouldn't make an invalid out of a person receiving chemotherapy treatment if that person is still able to function. Neither should the person who is sick be able to use his or her illness as a weapon, to ruin or control other people's lives. We are social animals who need some help, love, and reassurance from other people. But since family life gets emotionally complicated under the stress of medical treatment, do understand that you won't be the only person who will appreciate a little extra love and respect.

Remember that individuals have unique reactions to illness. Within the family, you may be able to find a particular person who can listen and comfort you in ways in which a professional cannot. Some relatives may withdraw for a time, but even if it hurts you a lot, try to allow them all the time they need to come around. Remember that family is always family. Whenever you feel like it, let people know that you're still the same person you were before being diagnosed with cancer—that you still have opinions, a point of view, and maybe even a sense of humor.

Friends

Friends can be another important source of support. Indeed, networks of friends have become much like an extended family for some people, especially many urban singles. As with family, you may have to make the first move to reestablish a relationship. Allow your friends some time to deal with their own feelings. When someone offers help, try to accept it. Some people really respond if you ask for something specific, and then politely thank them when they deliver. As with family, you may just lose some friends, through no fault of your own, simply because they are unable to deal with your illness and withdraw. Make sure you're not the one who is withdrawing from the friendship. If they don't call you, try picking up the phone once or twice and calling them before you write them off.

Co-Workers

Some people are comfortable discussing their chemotherapy at work, while others may bend over backward to make sure no one knows they've been ill because they are afraid someone will steal their job. Co-workers can be sympathetic; many people's lives have been touched by cancer. However, understand that most people don't want a blow-by-blow account of your illness. You will quickly lose even sympathetic listeners if every conversation involves a long, self-pitying speech about your medical condition. Be sensitive to other people's feelings, and use good judgment in this area. When in doubt, exercise caution.

How to Talk to Cancer Patients

Since you can be quite vulnerable when being treated for cancer, you may well experience a tremendous yearning for love, support, hope, and encouragement. Some people in your life won't have the first idea about how to meet these emotional needs. Even in these enlightened times, many people still don't know how to act, or even how to "just be themselves" when they encounter a person they know is undergoing chemotherapy. Harold Benjamin interviewed a group of people battling cancer and ex-cancer patients, and came up with the following tips for families and friends to use in talking to cancer patients:

1. Be natural—The person you see is the same person as before they got cancer. Benjamin believes that this is the absolute crux of the matter. Just because a person happens to come down with a disease, after all, doesn't mean that they suddenly become an alien from Mars. Your Aunt Emily is still your Aunt Emily, cancer or no cancer.
2. Don't avoid the subject of cancer and how it is affecting you. But first, ask if they mind discussing it.
3. Maintain regular contact with the cancer patient, and try to include them in your normal life.
4. Don't be afraid to show love or affection by touching them and hugging them, because they may feel very vulnerable and very unloved.
5. No pity allowed.
6. Don't tell cancer patients horror stories about other people with cancer or other diseases.
7. Share any success stories you hear about other people beating cancer.
8. Try to make yourself useful in a practical way.
9. Don't give medical advice unless you are asked. You might give the person articles or books to read, without telling them how to interpret the information.
10. Don't forget birthdays, anniversaries, and other more personal milestones such as the completion of chemotherapy.
11. Make the cancer patient a part of your life, much like before. Laugh together.
12. Don't try to set up a "we/they" situation. The patient is still your friend or your relative.

13. Don't expect the patient to die. Millions of people have already survived treatment for cancer.

Support Groups

If you're undergoing medical treatment, or dealing with someone who is, you may benefit from participation in a support group. Support groups are not the same as group counseling, although the structure is somewhat similar in that a number of people gather in a room at a particular time. Support groups are groups of people who are dealing with the effects of the same physical illness. People in support groups can be understanding about problems that you may not be able to discuss anywhere else. Where else are you going to find people who can crack jokes about cancer?

Harold Benjamin believes cancer patients need support groups because they are "abandoned both physically and emotionally by their family and friends, just when they need support the most." In the Los Angeles area, for instance, Wellness Community support groups are free to people being treated for cancer, or people whose cancer is in remission. Support groups can take many other forms.

Some hospital or community support groups are open to all cancer patients. Other support groups are targeted to particular people, such as women being treated for breast cancer, or spouses of men being treated for prostate cancer. Support groups such as the American Cancer Society's "I Can Cope" series may also be set up within a particular community. The American Cancer Society may also direct you to "one-on-one" programs that put you in contact with another person who has been through the same experience you have, sometimes through special "hot lines" that connect you with another person via the telephone. Groups such as the United Ostomy Association may be helpful in locating support groups for people who have had colostomies, ileostomies, or similar operations. Other specialized support groups exist.

Because support groups are composed of people living through the effects of cancer and cancer treatment, you may find it valuable to start or participate in a support group in your community. With a storm of powerful feelings in your heart, it can be very comforting to share your thoughts with another person or people who can appreciate how you feel, or even to listen to the concerns of other people. These days, it's no longer considered a sign of weakness to seek help. Although we are still a society that worships individualism, our attitudes toward support groups, Twelve Step programs, and other such "instant communities" have very definitely changed.

Support groups can sometimes meet certain play and recreational needs that often get lost in the course of treatment. Support groups can be a safe environment where participants know it's okay to laugh at an off-the-wall medical reference, or even joke about cancer. People in support groups can provide practical advice and referrals and help educate each other about various aspects of cancer treatment. The one point to understand about support groups is that they are all different. They vary according to who is participating in them at the time, and they are definitely not for everyone. Some social workers recommend that you sit in on a particular support group three times, and then decide whether participation is for you.

Janette's experience with support groups was admittedly "a disaster." She entered a support group at the hospital where she received chemotherapy. The group was composed of terminal liver cancer patients who seemed to be intent on "crying and dying," rather than "hoping and coping." She recalls, "It was depressing as hell." Janette quickly left the group and found her own way, which involved educating herself, sessions with a psychologist, and support from within her own warm circle of family and friends.

On-Line Support Groups

New technology is already making a wealth of medical information available to the general public, and the quantity of information is likely to increase. Some medical information can already be accessed via the World Wide Web, where the National Cancer

Institute and the American Cancer Society have home pages. The University of Iowa's "Virtual Hospital" Web page and other Internet addresses are included in the Other Resources appendix, although other electronic addresses are yet to appear. If you are proficient with computers, you'll soon have access to much of the medical information available in the world.

But beware of bad information, whatever the source. It is important to distinguish between actual support groups where you sit in a room with people whose faces you know, and ad hoc discussion groups where people type messages into their computers. When it comes to any on-line user group, computer bulletin board, or other electronic forum, cyberspace poses some particular problems in verifying information. The cyberphrase "information wants to be free" does not guarantee that a medical testimonial you receive from a person you can't identify is accurate. This type of electronic misinformation, unfortunately quite common, is discussed in chapter 19.

In short, you can't believe everything you hear. Even in an age of electronic and telecommunications miracles, consider the source of the medical information you receive. Your best and primary source of accurate medical information should remain your medical doctor.

Spiritual Resources

Interestingly, *therapeia,* the Greek root of the word "therapy," means "doing God's work." Local churches and synagogues are often an excellent source of help, since volunteers may be able to help you out at home in a number of practical and useful ways. When you're being treated for cancer, you may wish to renew your personal acquaintance with your minister or religious leader, because talking to that person can comfort you.

These days, spiritual care is part of the interdisciplinary approach being used in the best cancer treatment hospitals. The old chaplains who roamed the hospital with a Bible seeking to convert patients are pretty much a part of the past. Today, chaplains are sophisticated and well-trained people who respect your rights of privacy, but also make themselves available for counseling if you request it. Federal hospital accreditation requirements mandate that a chaplain be available to talk to patients twenty-four hours a day.

In comprehensive care hospitals, caregivers have observed that a great many people experience a sort of existential crisis during treatment. This long crisis is a process where the patient works through a storm of emotional pain to ultimately arrive at a peaceful acceptance of his or her own life and mortality. For many, this questioning and groping for answers has a profound spiritual dimension. While often painful to watch from the outside, this process can frequently leave patients with a new appreciation of their own life.

Most people have spiritual needs and spiritual passions, although not every person deals with them under the umbrella of an organized religion. Like Hans Castorp, the hero of Thomas Mann's classic novel, *The Magic Mountain,* everyone finds his or her own way to move through an illness and continue on with life.

Working through this personal crisis can deepen a loving relationship. A woman with breast cancer may fear rejection by her partner after treatment has changed her physical appearance, but ultimately be relieved and grateful to find herself accepted by her partner for who she is rather than her body image alone.

It is a rarely acknowledged upside of cancer treatment that many, many people come through the physical and emotional turmoil with a new understanding and a profound appreciation of daily life. After the storm has passed, family ties may strengthen. Children may have actually or finally risen to the occasion, accepting more responsibility than ever before. Parents of children with cancer may feel grateful for the good care given to their beloved child.

Things important enough to argue about before the diagnosis of cancer may not seem so important after this crisis has passed. You may learn that it is not *what you do* that defines you, but rather *who you are.* You may reflect on the words of author Robert Louis Stevenson, who once observed, "Life is not a matter of holding good cards, but of playing a poor hand well."

Several years ago in the *New England Journal of Medicine,* Robert M. Mack, a surgeon, wrote down what recovering from cancer meant to him: "I am very grateful just to be alive. I am very glad to have been permitted to learn to live with, rather than simply die from, my cancer. Mostly, I am glad to measure my life not in terms of what it once was or what I might have wished it to be but in terms of how wonderful it is now. I am glad to recognize each day as a splendid, unforgettable miracle, a wonderful gift for me to savor and enjoy as fully as I can."

As you have seen, you may draw emotional support from a network of many people, including friends, family members, co-workers, counselors, social workers, and people you meet in support groups. All may help support you in some way. Indeed, on the most profound level of your being, you may move through chemotherapy and discover what's actually most important in your life.

Chemotherapy treatment has many aspects, not the least of which are practical aspects. Some of the most important practical details you must address are financial—the topic of the next chapter of this book.

18

MONEY ISSUES

DEALING WITH THE
COSTS OF CHEMOTHERAPY

CHEMOTHERAPY COSTS MONEY. UNDERSTANDING HOW TO BEST APPROACH the financial aspects of chemotherapy, and how to locate and utilize other sources of financial help, is the topic of this chapter. Included are suggestions for resolving payment problems with health insurance companies, and finding new health insurance and other types of help when you need it.

Expenses for chemotherapy drugs alone can range in cost from $20 to $100 per cycle to as much as $1,000 per cycle. Drugs classified as "investigational," which have not been FDA-approved, may be given free of cost if they are part of a clinical study. But manufacturers may also legally bill for investigational drugs if certain conditions regarding their use are met.

A year of chemotherapy can easily cost from $3,000 to $20,000 or more. What you pay depends on a number of factors including the number of treatments, the anticancer drug or drugs employed, and whether you must be hospitalized or may be treated as an outpatient. As a point of reference, six months' adjuvant therapy for breast cancer might cost from $3,000 to $5,000. A year of chemotherapy for colon cancer might cost $5,000 to $6,000. Chemotherapy treatments with the more expensive platinum-based drugs, which must always be given in a hospital, might cost

$3,000 per treatment including hospital costs, or upwards of $20,000 for six treatments. Other treatment modalities such as surgery involve additional costs, of course, as do medical tests and procedures.

According to one survey of cancer treatment at a health maintenance organization in the state of Washington, pictured here in the chart on page 201, the average cost of the first six months of treatment (using all modalities) for prostate, breast, or colon cancer ranged from $9,000 to $15,000.

The costs of hospital care alone range from an average of $1,300 per day in an urban area to an average cost of $800 a day in a rural area. Incidental costs such as transportation and child care can increase the financial burden of cancer to you.

In the United States, whether you're covered by health insurance or not, you have a right to have a detailed estimate of the cost of your treatment before you begin. You may request this estimate in writing, if your doctor does not offer it to you right away, for inclusion in your medical file.

Chemotherapy is covered at least in part by most health insurance policies, including Medicare Part B, which covers 80 percent of what the federal government considers to be reasonable medical services such as outpatient hospital care, diagnostic tests, and administered drugs. In some states, chemotherapy is covered under Medicaid. Ideally, your health insurance policy will cover all of the cost of chemotherapy although it is more likely it will cover only certain portions of the costs.

Even if you don't have health insurance, several sources of help listed later in this chapter may be of use to you and your family in handling some of the expenses you will incur.

Health Insurance

Dealing with a health insurance company can be quite frustrating for the average person, but experts advise working through problems and documenting your concerns in a professional manner. If payment for a claim is denied, don't assume that to be a definitive

COSTS OF CHEMOTHERAPY DRUGS

High Cost
($500 to $1,000 and up per cycle)
carboplatin, cisplatin, estramustine, interferon, interleukin-2,
leuprolide, mitomycin

Medium Cost
($100 to $500 per cycle)
asparaginase, bleomycin, carmustine, cytarabine,
dacarbazine, daunorubicin, dactinomycin, doxorubicin,
etoposide, floxuridine, ifosfamide, leucovorin, lomustine,
melphalan, mercaptopurine, methotrexate, mitotane,
mitoxantrone, plicamycin, streptozocin, tamoxifen, thiotepa,
vinblastine, vincristine

Low Cost
($20 to $100 per cycle)
busulfan, chlorambucil, cyclophosphamide, fluorouracil,
mechlorethamine, prednisone, procarbazine

AVERAGE COSTS OF CANCER CARE

Cancer	Initial Care	Continuing Care	Terminal Care
Breast	$10,813	$1,084	$17,686
Colon	$14,968	$1,318	$12,110
Prostate	$9,060	$1,379	$15,551

Initial care indicates first six months of care; terminal care indicates last six months of life. This information is taken from a study of cancer costs in a Washington State HMO, published in the Journal of the National Cancer Institute, *March 15, 1995. Costs of chemotherapy and other treatment modalities are combined.*

answer. Continue to try to collect the payment, and build a case as to why you feel you are entitled to payment. Most people do get paid eventually, although it can take a long time, anywhere from eight weeks to nine months.

You might want to start a financial records file, where you keep all your medical records and insurance records in one location, such as a box or a desk drawer. When you speak to a person at your insurance company, write down who you speak to, when you spoke to them, and what they told you. Include this in your file. Keep these records in one notebook or file where you can find this information when you need it. Keep copies of your letters to insurance companies, and their responses to your letters in the file. If you don't feel well, perhaps you can ask a spouse or a trusted friend to help you keep up this paperwork. Keeping good financial records files is useful even if you don't have health insurance. Having access to your records will allow you to present a stronger case if you have to argue with an insurance company or anyone else over financial issues.

Doctors find it frustrating when insurance companies try to limit their choice of therapies to those that cost less, rather than those that are most effective. According to one Gallup survey of cancer doctors, from 15 to 40 percent of their patients had been denied the treatment of choice by insurance companies. Insurance companies won't pay for treatments they consider "experimental." In some instances, insurance companies are simply not aware of newer and more effective cancer treatments, and they may not wish to pay for them unless information about the effectiveness of treatments is provided to them and they accept the rationale. If you must go through this process of providing information that will prove the effectiveness of your treatment, take heart in knowing that you may make it slightly easier for the next person who comes along. If your doctors say you need a life-saving treatment and your insurance doesn't want to cover it, take the treatment and argue with your insurance company later.

All anticancer drugs come with a "package insert" listing its dosages for particular types of cancer. However, new treatments are being developed so rapidly that experts estimate that about *half* the average anticancer drug's approved and effective uses in cancer treatment are *not* given on the package inserts. Groups such as the Association of Community Cancer Centers are working to pass laws requiring insurance companies to pay for off-label uses of particular drugs that have been proven to extend and improve the quality of patients' lives.

Today, not all insurance plans are alike. You can't always choose your own doctor. Early on, find out exactly what your health insurance plan covers. Some insurance plans such as Blue Cross will more fully cover payments to an oncologist who participates in their plan. Health maintenance organizations will probably want you to be treated by a particular oncologist or will restrict your choices to a small group.

Note that it is your responsibility to be sure that you receive the maximum benefits your plan allows. If you assume that a particular service is covered by your insurance and later find out it is not, in most cases you are responsible to pay for the service and you will receive a bill. Likewise, if you do not submit a claim for a service that is covered by your policy, you may not be reimbursed even if you discover your mistake and notify the insurance company. Often the insurance company's decision whether or not to reimburse depends upon how much time has lapsed since the date of treatment and the date the claim is filed.

Some health insurance companies do pay for items such as hospital beds or prostheses, but they don't put this information in their informational brochures, or they reduce it to easily overlooked fine print. To verify benefits such as these, speak with the customer service department of your insurance company. Before you begin treatment you can usually request a preauthorization of benefits, which the insurance company will provide. Preauthorization explains what portion of your anticipated treatment costs is covered by your policy.

Some costs are almost never covered by insurance, such as parents' travel to and from hospitals for a child with cancer. For tax purposes, keep a record and receipts for all your health-related expenses, even transportation and lodging, because expenses not reimbursed by insurance may be tax deductible.

Insurance Survival Tips

Here are some tips on dealing with insurance companies:

- Make sure your premiums are paid up to date.
- Ask for and then study a copy of the most recent plan booklet from your insurance carrier.
- Check your policy to see if you have a "waiver of premium" feature that allows you to pay no premiums during your time of treatment or disability.
- Get a supply of blank insurance claim forms.
- Make copies of all forms you submit, and make copies of all correspondence between you and the insurance company including letters and faxes.
- Make sure that you understand all the benefits that are available under your policy and that you receive all the coverage to which you are entitled.
- If you speak to a person over the telephone at your insurance company, ask for and write down that person's name and include it in your medical records file.
- Submit claims for everything for which you are billed, including wigs and medicine.
- Review your bills for accuracy, and report the errors that do occur.

If you are treated at a hospital or clinic that will supply the anticancer drugs and bill the insurance companies directly, you'll save on out-of-pocket costs. If you must buy chemotherapy drugs from pharmacies, call both chain and nonchain drugstores and compare costs. Some pharmacies are now associated with particular insurance plans and will supply drugs at the lowest cost.

In the case of an item you might consider vitally necessary, such as a hairpiece or wig, you might ask your doctor to write a prescription for a *hair prosthesis*. When you purchase the wig, have the receipt state that it is for a hair prosthesis, and not a wig or hairpiece. Getting written documentation is often helpful in your being reimbursed by insurance companies, who have guidelines they must follow for reimbursement.

In the case of special equipment you might need for a period of time, such as hospital beds you need for home care, you might compare the costs of renting this equipment against purchasing it outright. Insurance company representatives should also be consulted, since companies vary in which of these costs they will reimburse, and you should know this going in. Calling a few recommended suppliers and companies listed in the yellow pages will get you the most competitive prices for these items.

Payment Problems

If your claim for payment has been denied, have your doctor's office double-check the bill to make sure the correct procedure code and diagnosis has been written on the insurance claim. If that isn't the problem, make your doctors and their office staff aware of your situation. The doctor's office may be able to query the insurer, and to provide further information about your treatment regimen if that is needed to process a claim.

Get on the phone if you have a problem with your insurance company. If the first person with whom you speak can't or won't help you, ask to speak with that person's supervisor. Work your way right up to the president of the company if you feel like your problem is very important. You may also demand answers to your questions by writing letters or sending faxes.

Ask your insurance company to review any claim in question. Most companies have a procedure to review claims, and customer service representatives at your insurance company can explain this procedure to you over the telephone. Your oncologist's office staff can also often consult with the drug company that manufactures the anticancer drugs you have received. If your medical oncologist requests it, the drug manufacturer might be able to provide further information to the insurance company to help get your claim paid. Some reimbursement specialists are located at "hot lines" maintained by drug companies—these people can sometimes help you obtain payment by searching the literature for pertinent research data, or even by directly contacting insurers. Tell your doctor about these people, whose services are free.

Insurance companies are certified by individual states, not by the federal government. Cancer organizations in many states are working to educate decision makers at insurance companies about new treatments, and to set minimum insurance standards for cancer treatment—something that needs to be done.

Lawsuits are definitely a last resort, but sometimes the only way to secure payment for a disputed claim or to resolve a disputed issue. Individuals have prevailed in court over insurance companies, or discriminatory policies. As an example, one athletic young man who had beaten testicular cancer two years previously applied for his dream job with the local police department, only to be denied because of his medical history. The police department's policy required that applicants be free of cancer for five years, but this was patently illegal. The young man got an attorney at legal aid to take his case, and eventually got the department's hiring policy overturned. Happily, he got his job on the force—with five years' seniority, back pay, legal fees, and compensatory damages. However, keep in mind the majority of civil lawsuits end up without a clear winner, with both sides paying legal fees.

COBRA

Think twice before you quit a job that has good health insurance if a member of your family is chronically ill. Insurance companies consider people who have recovered from cancer "high risk." The Medical Information Bureau (MIB), located in Boston, Massachusetts, collects and shares medical information on individuals with more than seven-hundred commercial insurance carriers, excluding Blue Cross and Blue Shield. Every medical detail of almost every application you've submitted for health insurance in the past seven years ends up in the MIB database.

What insurance companies call "preexisting conditions" can make getting more health insurance coverage difficult or expensive. An insurance company can put limits called "impairment exclusion" riders on the kinds of medical care that new policies will cover. For instance, you might be offered medical coverage at the regular rate, which covers every kind of illness except cancer. Or you might have to pay extra to receive coverage for cancer.

"My insurance plan covered almost everything when I was treated for cancer, and I was lucky," said one man who beat cancer five years ago, but who has since switched careers and insurance companies. "But let me tell you—I have to pay a *lot* of money for insurance coverage now."

If you quit a job that provided you health insurance, and you worked for a company with twenty or more employees, your employer is required to offer you and your dependents the option of continuing the coverage for eighteen months, with you paying the entire premium. This is called COBRA coverage, after a federal law called the Consolidated Omnibus Budget Reconciliation Act of 1985. If you get new insurance, you are required to relinquish your COBRA policy unless your new policy is limited or carries a preexisting condition clause. In this case, you may continue your coverage under COBRA to cover the waiting period required by your new insurance.

If COBRA doesn't apply to you, you might be able to convert your former employer's group policy to one that covers you as an individual or family. You may seek the services of an insurance broker who specializes in finding insurance for high-risk people. You may be able to secure health insurance through a trade association or professional group. The American Association of Retired Persons (better known as AARP), for instance, offers health plans to their members who are age fifty or over. Some health maintenance organizations have "open enrollment" periods during which they will accept anyone who wishes to join up. More than a dozen states also have "risk pools" of health insurance, which will insure anyone regardless of their medical history.

If you are seeking insurance and have been denied coverage from your job, private insurance companies, HMOs, or other sources and feel you have been treated unfairly, your state department of insurance may be able to help if you file a complaint.

Hospital Patients

Many hospitals have a department called patient finances or patient accounts, which collects money for hospital services.

People who work in these departments will work with your insurance company. Unless the insurance company has flatly refused to pay the hospital, or you have no insurance coverage, patient finances people will probably not ask you for the entire cost of the hospital stay. These people can sometimes be persuaded to allow you to pay your bill in installments, or help you apply for government aid if you need it.

If you can't pay a particular bill, or if you feel a bill is incorrect, stop by the patient finances department or call them to discuss the problem. Explain your problem with the bill, and insist on payment arrangements that you can live with. Ask for a patient representative or a social worker if you cannot resolve this issue by yourself.

If you receive chemotherapy as an outpatient in a private medical oncologist's office, note that doctors have office managers or particular employees who specialize in billing. If you have a problem with a bill, speak with this person first. If you don't resolve the problem with the office manager's help, ask to speak with the doctor.

Other Sources of Help

If you can't work, you may be able to receive payment from your employer's disability insurance policy. In addition, you may qualify for state government disability payments to help replace your income. Although the laws may change, Medicare is currently available to some men and women under the age of sixty-five who have cancer and who are disabled. You have the right to appeal decisions that deny you disability payments from Social Security or Medicaid.

Any military veteran is eligible for free medical treatment in a Veterans Administration hospital. Merchant Marine veterans or

Native Americans may be treated free of charge at a public health service hospital.

If you need help paying for chemotherapy treatments, the local office of the American Cancer Society or the Cancer Information Service may be able to direct you to other sources of financial help. Organizations such as the Leukemia Society of America have programs that will help people with certain types of cancer who are in need of financial help. Some drug companies have programs that will pay the cost of their company's chemotherapy drugs for patients who have no other way to pay. A few sources of financial help are listed in the Other Resources appendix of this book.

At the National Cancer Institute in Bethesda, Maryland, treatment is free. Some of the major teaching hospitals offer treatment in a clinic setting. These institutions will frequently adjust fees on a sliding scale, or accept what insurance you have. Some comprehensive cancer treatment hospitals have only experimental therapy available for some types of cancer, although standard treatment may be available for most. Clinical research trials, which cover the costs of treatment, may sometimes be an option the first time around, or if the first round of chemotherapy isn't effective. Consult with your medical oncologist before participating in a clinical trial, and locate one with some chance for helping people with your type and stage of cancer.

Other Concerns

Even if you are not wealthy, a financial advisor found via referral from your bank or broker can counsel you on the best way to invest your money or organize your finances during the time when you are undergoing chemotherapy and beyond. As a general rule, you will probably not wish to place your money in nonliquid, volatile, or risky types of investments during this time because they can take a long time to sell or lose a lot of their value in a short period of time. You may need to tap into your investments without much notice.

You may incur heavy expenses, some of which you cannot anticipate, during treatment for your illness. Bankruptcy may be an option in some extreme situations, if medical bills are overwhelming and you have no means of repaying them.

In dealing with the ramifications of chemotherapy treatment, you may also wish to consult with an attorney. An attorney can help you in cases of bankruptcy, job discrimination, and medical malpractice. An attorney can help you draw up a will. As a precaution you may want to prepare a living will, a legal document that prohibits "heroic" measures to keep you alive when your chances of surviving are effectively gone. At some point during your medical treatment, you may want to consider giving a trusted friend or relative power of attorney so that he or she can sign checks for you in case you are unable to do so. If you change your mind, your power of attorney can be withdrawn.

Chemotherapy treatments will affect your finances. But know that you are not powerless in the financial area. If you have health insurance, you can solve most of the difficulties you encounter with health insurance claims, or you can seek help resolving these problems. In some cases, other options for covering the costs of chemotherapy are available to you.

It is important to discriminate between good medical treatment and the medical quackery touched upon in the next chapter. Unorthodox cancer cures look good at first glance, but they are never reimbursed by insurance for one good reason—they usually don't work.

19

UNORTHODOX THERAPIES

BEWARE THE MIRACLE CURE

EACH YEAR, THOUSANDS OF PEOPLE EXPERIMENT WITH UNORTHODOX or unproven treatment therapies for cancer that don't actually affect their disease and could be truly harmful. This chapter explains why some of these remedies are attractive, lists a few of the treatments, and explains why oftentimes they should be avoided. If you feel you should try an unorthodox therapy, this chapter offers suggestions for combining it with conventional medical care, under your doctor's supervision.

Unorthodox treatments for cancer are those that occur outside the wide range of mainstream medicine and that have not been scientifically proven to control cancer. We are not referring to *alternative* care or stress-relieving techniques, such as those listed in chapter 16, which are completely legitimate and whose use is often encouraged by doctors to supplement medical treatment. We are talking about *unorthodox* or bogus medicine that, in and of itself, does not cure cancer.

A prime example of this is laetrile, a product made from the pits of apricots, which was widely touted as a miracle cure for cancer in the late 1970s. Lots of legitimate newspapers, magazines, and television newscasts ran stories about laetrile, suggesting this unorthodox treatment might be the new miracle cure for cancer. Eventually, the National Cancer Institute completed scientific studies, including the special diets recommended to be followed with treatment, and the research showed laetrile to be medically worthless. Actor Steve McQueen was one of the many people who tried laetrile and found it did not cure his cancer.

Barrie R. Cassileth, Ph.D., has studied unorthodox treatments and written that *legitimate* treatment methods will meet all the following criteria:

1. The method was studied scientifically, and shown to be more effective than no treatment at all.
2. The benefits of the method are greater than the harm it might do.
3. Studies of the method have been conducted in a proper scientific manner, designed properly, and subjected to a review by their peers or others in the field. Studies involving human beings must be reviewed and approved by the human subjects committee of an established, reputable medical institution.

Most unorthodox treatments claim to be miracle cures, but aren't. A few may have helped a few people a few times. But unorthodox cancer treatments can be quite dangerous if they are substituted for medically proven treatments such as chemotherapy, which have been scientifically proven to control or cure cancer. Looked at rationally, it stands to reason that if the treatment you receive has no effect on your tumor, cancer cells will continue to grow and spread in your body, and eventually disable a vital organ, which will cause your death.

Every oncologist has seen patients leave their care to take a miracle cure, which delayed legitimate medical treatment, and then seen those same patients come back after so much time had passed that they had reduced or eliminated their chance of achieving a remission.

Unorthodox methods of treating cancer include multiple enemas, megavitamin therapy, unusual substances like laetrile, or special diets. Many, many unproven therapies involve manipulations of the normal diet far beyond the realm of good nutrition. Unorthodox practitioners add to the confusion by billing themselves as "natural" or "holistic" or "alternative," legitimate words that disguise the truly worthless nature of their treatments. Some practitioners claim they "clean out the toxins" from the body by various means, such as multiple enemas with various substances such as coffee. Some recent fads include claims that substances such as shark cartilage, wheat grass, or Kombucha mushrooms can cure cancer, claims that are scientifically unproven.

Work with Your Doctor

Because there's been such an explosion of interest in nutrition and good health over the past several years, some oncologists encourage their patients to pursue most alternative treatments, as long as they do it simultaneously with a legitimate treatment for cancer such as chemotherapy and keep the doctor apprised. A study published in the *New England Journal of Medicine* estimated as many as one-third of patients try an unconventional therapy, usually as an adjunct to conventional therapy, but most did not share this information with their physician. Special diets and vitamin supplements are approved by many physicians if substances are not taken in dangerous amounts. Several programs package several nonmedical elements together, but insist on medical support. For instance, the Commonweal Cancer Help program in San Francisco utilizes yoga, meditation, deep relaxation and imagery, massage therapy, work with sand trays, and a vegetarian diet in their program, which is designed to enhance the quality of life of cancer patients. But this program—and other legitimate programs designed to help cancer patients—require that people who participate also be under the care of an oncologist.

Dr. Bernie Siegel has advised physicians, "If people are doing things outside your belief system, accept them and love them, even if you don't agree with their choices. In that way patients will feel comfortable and cared for by the medical profession and be able to make use of all the options available to them. They can tolerate disagreement, but not destructiveness."

Many oncologists feel it is important to give patients a sense of control and participation in the healing process. But any oncologist would warn his or her patients against practices and methods that could be medically dangerous. And, unfortunately, some oncologists are downright hostile to methods that don't neatly fit under the umbrella of conventional medicine.

"One Size Fits All"

Important differences exist between medical doctors and laypeople who treat diseases with unproven techniques. Typically, unorthodox practitioners use exactly the same miracle cure on everybody, regardless of the type and stage of the cancer. Most don't establish that you have cancer with a biopsy, which in almost every case is the only medically certain way to diagnose it. Many of these types of practitioners are charismatic people who actually believe that their treatments can work, while others are just opportunists cynically cashing in on people's hopes, with no illusions about the value of their treatments. Many of these types of practitioners claim that they are persecuted by the cancer "establishment," which is "out to get them" because they have a secret cure that nobody else wants to use because it's inexpensive and doesn't need to be administered by a medical doctor. This plays into a general distrust of institutions many people already have.

Beware of these very seductive "cancer cures" that promise to cure you without any physical pain or discomfort, without tests, without surgery, without radiation, without chemotherapy, without hospital care, and without side effects. These kinds of promises are incredibly attractive to people who dread the so-called "cut, burn, and poison" stereotypes of cancer treatment. Even sophisticated people who are curious and well-read often don't know of all the advances that cancer treatment has made in the past several years. Unfortunately, the wish for a "magic bullet" to cure cancer is so seductive and so powerful that it leads thousands of people down blind alleys every year.

The average person encounters a lot of information every day. With all the medical factoids in the air, and half-truths blithely reported in the media as "medical breakthroughs," it's admittedly a big task to sort through all the competing claims. Cancer quacks can add smoke and noise to the medical confusion.

Quackery Travels Fast

These days, claims of miracle cures can be made and disseminated by the electronic media in the twinkling of an eye, yet take years of clinical trial research to disprove. Within our very news-intensive society, the focus is most often on the new and sensational, rather the accurate and boring. As a result, medical misinformation is distributed faster than ever before.

Lately, a lot of medical misinformation has begun to move over the Internet. Misinformation is sometimes being exchanged via holistic health chat groups on computer on-line services, according to physicians who have monitored these on-line discussions. To protect yourself, be wary of testimonials by people who claim to have been cured by this or that unorthodox method, such as an exotic herb, vitamin, or mushroom. In the end, a lot of people trumpeting unorthodox medical products over the Internet simply have a financial interest in selling them.

Already, Internet addresses and World Wide Web home pages have been established by people peddling questionable treatments. Since *we all* enjoy the right of freedom of speech, it can be difficult for medical consumers to distinguish between real and false information. Behind impressively designed home pages, some of these practitioners cloak themselves in legitimacy by providing home page referrals to legitimate medical organizations. In cyberspace, legitimate organizations such as the American Cancer Society can have a home page, but so can Kombucha mushrooms.

One medical doctor with an interest in the Internet tells the tragic story of a teenage boy who got AIDS through a blood transfusion. The boy was given a computer by his parents. The young man learned how to use the computer, poked around the Internet, and found an unorthodox practitioner in Tijuana, Mexico, who treated AIDS with a very questionable treatment involving electric shocks. Before they could be persuaded otherwise, the young man and his parents traveled to Tijuana and spent a lot of money for electric shock treatment, which is medically worthless and could not cure his AIDS.

Instant Gratification

Since we are a society that seeks instant gratification, we are particularly vulnerable to modern-day snake-oil salesmen who promise quick, painless cancer cures. According to one study, many people choose these unorthodox therapies mainly to avoid the side effects of conventional medical treatment and not because they have an advanced case of cancer that can't be cured. It is not against the law for adults to try *any* treatment method. For children with cancer, however, the courts have generally held that it's illegal for parents to select unproven methods.

Unorthodox treatment clinics do often treat their patients with lots of warmth and affection, something lacking in many doctors' offices. The costs of an unorthodox treatment could be less than you might spend for conventional treatment, although none of your money would be reimbursed by health insurance. And it probably would not work.

The promise of a painless, instant, New Age cure is much more compelling than a skeptical doctor's hard, mathematical assessment of your chances for survival, especially if the doctor includes an explanation of possible side effects. The plain truth is, only good medicine can offer you reasonable hope for survival.

Participate Carefully

It is extremely beneficial to participate in your own healing, particularly when you use some of the legitimate, proven methods outlined in chapter 16 of this book. But do be skeptical of so-called secret cures, which are often kept secret because they won't stand up to scrutiny by other medical professionals. Reputable organizations such as the American Cancer Society and the National Cancer Institute maintain data banks of information about unproven treatments for cancer, and some other organizations keep track of fraudulent cancer treatments and issue position papers on many of them. If you have any questions about an unusual or unorthodox cancer treatment, check first using references listed in the Other Resources appendix of this book.

Unorthodox cancer treatments should be avoided because they don't work and could be dangerous. If you wish to participate in your treatment with something like a special diet, please do so with the full knowledge of your oncologist. Take a hand in your own treatment. If you are careful not to damage your own health, the benefits of positive action are considerable. Just don't forsake good medical treatment. Despite some drawbacks, treatments like chemotherapy still offer you the best possible chance for extending the length and quality of your life.

Some happy day, as you'll learn in the subsequent chapter, your chemotherapy treatments may be complete. At that time, with a clean bill of health, you'll be ready to move on with your life.

20

BEYOND CHEMOTHERAPY

WHEN YOUR TREATMENT IS OVER

WHAT DO YOU DO WHEN CHEMOTHERAPY IS FINALLY OVER? YOU'LL probably want to follow a more healthy lifestyle to lessen the chances of cancer recurring. You'll have no shortage of other related issues to deal with in your life, including continuing medical checkups, work, and lifestyle issues, which include adjustments for you and those around you.

Breathe a big sigh of relief when you finish chemotherapy treatments. But understand, too, that it's very normal to fear a recurrence of cancer after chemotherapy treatments have stopped. In fact, the period after chemotherapy can be a very stressful period of time, because many people get very anxious each time they must return to their medical oncologist for a checkup.

People who have had cancer are at a slightly higher risk of developing a second cancer than people who have never had cancer. Certainly, these statistics vary depending on the type of cancer and other medical factors. It won't do to enter a state of psychological denial and avoid returning to the doctor's office at all. Although you probably didn't enjoy chemotherapy, you can't just turn tail and run at the smell of rubbing alcohol or the sight of butterfly IVs. Further tests are necessary. You'll need to arrive at a realistic assessment of the chances that you might have a recurrence—neither denying the possibility a second cancer could occur, or exaggerating the risks involved.

Second incidences of cancer are not that frequent. They occur in only between 5 to 10 percent of all chemotherapy patients. Most commonly, second malignancies occur at least three years after treatment. The most common time to see a recurrence is seven to ten years after chemotherapy, although this varies according to the type of cancer and other factors. Ask your physician to assess the chances of your suffering a recurrence.

Here are two things you can do which will probably increase your life span after chemotherapy treatments:

- Have regular checkups as recommended by your doctor.
- Live a healthy lifestyle.

Even if you feel great, you may experience anxiety and fear in the pit of your stomach every time you are called back into your doctor's office for tests to monitor your progress. But you will probably heave a huge sigh of relief when your tests show no new cancer. Remember that even if you do have a recurrence, the frequent checkups will make it possible to catch it at a very early stage when the chances of a cure are highest.

One man whose cancer was in remission found it much easier to visit the doctor's office when he reminded himself he was there as a visitor, not as a patient. Others find it helpful to take another person along to the doctor's office.

At some point, your oncologist may tell you that you are past the danger point for a recurrence. Five years is a rule of thumb for most types of cancer, but the period of greatest medical wariness varies considerably and can be either more or less than five years. Still, for most types of cancer, being in remission for five years, or past the point of greatest danger, is a very healthy sign.

A Changed Life

Your life may not just neatly fall back into place after medical treatment is over, as many people have learned.

Although Susan Nessim was diagnosed with cancer at the age

of seventeen, good medical treatment helped her defeat a rare cancer, rhabdomyosarcoma, within about a year. She found it difficult to leave her experience with cancer behind her. She was humiliated when she was rejected by her fiancé's family because of her medical condition. She was stunned when she was aced out of a promotion at a large cosmetics company by a co-worker who whispered to her boss that her medical condition would not allow her to perform all the travel necessary for the job. Nine years after being cured of cancer, Susan looked for a support group and found only groups for patients currently undergoing treatment. Seeing and feeling the need to begin a support group system for cancer survivors, she started an organization called Cancervive, which is now headquartered in Los Angeles with several branches nation-wide.

Many people say a period of social adjustment or even up-heaval is not unusual, even after the cancer has been driven into remission. A co-founder of the National Coalition for Cancer Survivorship, Fitzhugh Mullan, M.D., named this condition "the Humpty Dumpty syndrome." Like the character in that famous old nursery rhyme who had a great fall, as a survivor you try to pick up all the pieces of your life and put them together again. The truth is, the pieces of your life may not fit together in exactly the same way they fit together before.

For one thing, cancer survivors often see the world differently after they recover. Your family and friends who steeled them-selves for the worst now have to adjust to the idea that you're back in their lives and that your needs may be a bit different than they were before. If you have young children, they may expect you to automatically become the same old mommy or daddy you were before your cancer diagnosis, even if you're not completely re-covered from the effects of chemotherapy. Children who have been treated for cancer may expect a lot more attention. Spouses or friends who have patiently stood by your side may feel like they've "done their part," and react to any additional needs you have with anger or resentment . . . in a few cases, these people just pack their suitcases and walk out the door. In some families, the reaction is a kind of collective denial—to insist on acting like "everything is just fine," whether everything is actually fine or not. On the other side of the coin, your friends or relatives may overindulge you, pampering you and overprotecting you as if you're still sick when you're no longer really a sick person at all.

Communication

In all these situations and many more, communication is the key to striking a balance between you and the people who surround you. If you think you have a problem, start by telling the other person exactly how *you* feel about the situation without laying blame or guilt on them. Start your sentences with "I feel . . . ," then give the other person a chance to respond and listen carefully to what he or she has to say. Time heals emotional wounds. Give yourself and your family and friends time to make the adjustment, because such issues are not resolved overnight. Think of yourself as a survivor rather than a victim, and take positive action to improve your life.

New acquaintances may have either good or bad reactions to the news that you are recovering from cancer. If you're a single person, you may find yourself rejected by a potential lover who just can't accept the idea that you have been seriously ill. This can be temporarily devastating. In other cases, you may form a deep bond with individuals who have had some experience with serious illness in their own lives or seen the effects of illness on the lives of people they have loved dearly in their own families. Understand that your own attitude about your recovery from cancer will affect how people react to you. Learn to love and value yourself, and try to do the same for others. Remember that Mother Teresa stated that the greatest disease afflicting the human race is simply the absence of love.

Good Health

Practicing a healthy lifestyle will help you stave off recurrences of cancer. Eat a nutritious diet rich with fruits and vegetables containing adequate vitamins A, C, and E, which may help prevent

the return of cancer. At minimum, follow the same dietary recommendations made by the American Cancer Society for all people, which are listed in chapter 12—generally a high-fiber, low-fat
diet containing at least five servings per day of fruits and vegetables. Work to control your weight, because obesity is a risk factor
for cancer.

Similar risk factors apply to people who have had cancer as to
those who have not. According to *Everyone's Guide to Cancer
Therapy,* of the two largest identified risk factors, diet is believed
to play a role in 30 to 35 percent of cancers, and the use of tobacco
to play a role in 30 to 32 percent of cancers. Your use of alcohol,
your exposure to chemical carcinogens, your exposure to sunlight,
and even your personal and family medical history are documented risk factors for cancer.

You'll reduce your risk of a recurrence if you clean up your
diet, stop smoking, and reduce your use of alcoholic beverages to
modest amounts.

Moderate exercise strengthens your body, of course. Exercise
helps rejuvenate your immune system after it has been weakened
by chemotherapy. Exercise has cardiovascular and many other
well-known benefits—including a possible link with the prevention of some types of cancers such as breast cancer. And don't forget to exercise your mind, by learning about new things or
pursuing interests that are important to you.

Some individuals just refuse to be denied what they seek in
life. If you think your life is over because you've had cancer, look
at Jeff Blatnik, an athlete who was diagnosed with Hodgkin's disease in 1982. Two years later, Blatnik won a gold medal for
wrestling at the Los Angeles Olympic Games.

Certainly, your mind and your body work together to achieve
good mental and physical health. Two hundred Harvard
University undergraduates were questioned before World War II,
and every year thereafter as they moved through their lives in the
postwar era. Those judged to have the best mental health lived
much longer and with less disease than those whose mental
health was worse.

Work Life

Some people never stop working when they have chemotherapy treatments, while others must take some time off from work for treatments and recovery. As you begin to cycle back into a more normal life, you may have to begin your activities slowly, because your body is weak. Build up strength and endurance on the job. If you work at it, you'll soon see an improvement. It helps, of course, if you have a sympathetic employer who really likes you and who values your work.

It is a myth that employees who have survived cancer are less productive than other employees, although some employers continue to believe it. More than twenty years ago, studies by AT&T and the Metropolitan Life Insurance Company tracked the work histories of employees who had recovered from cancer. About 80 percent of the AT&T employees who were treated for cancer returned to their jobs, and performed as long and as well as other employees. The Metropolitan study found no difference in absenteeism, turnover, or work performance between cancer survivors and the control group. Metropolitan concluded that hiring employees who had survived cancer was "sound industrial practice."

Despite research results that prove people who have survived cancer are good employees, your own work life could still take a turn for the worse. Discrimination at work is a sensitive issue, and it occurs. Cancer is considered a legal disability. People who have had cancer are legally protected against discrimination on the job through the federal Americans with Disabilities Act (ADA) of 1990, and through the Federal Rehabilitation Act of 1973. All states have passed laws against discriminating against people who are handicapped, although not every state's laws include cancer survivors in their definition of handicapped. The American Civil Liberties Union, which has offices in most major cities, is a source of legal assistance for people who feel they have been victimized by discrimination.

The ADA prohibits an employer from firing you based solely on the fact that you were treated for cancer. The ADA also protects people who have been treated for cancer against discrimination in hiring, promotions, transfers, and layoffs. There is some anecdotal evidence that people who have been treated for cancer are discriminated against after they have been cured, by being shunted off into dead-end jobs and by not getting a chance to be promoted again. Observers speculate that employers may believe that they are driving up their health insurance costs by having an employee with cancer and may fear the financial consequences if the person comes down with cancer again. These fears are rarely verbalized, but can have a powerful effect on your career no matter what your actual performance. Subtle discrimination is difficult but not impossible to prove.

And since finding a job with good health insurance is more difficult after you've been treated for cancer, some people fall into a condition called "job lock," where they remain working for a company with a good insurance plan even if they have to take a demotion or stay in a job they have outgrown. New jobs with good insurance are not impossible to find. As a general rule, you will be more easily accepted into a large company's insurance plan than a small company's plan if you have a history of cancer. Large companies have a larger pool of patients to insure, so they are less concerned about one person's health problems driving up their insurance premiums.

Other resources are patient advocacy groups with information on insurance and employment discrimination against cancer patients. One of these is the National Coalition for Cancer Survivorship, whose address and telephone number may be found in the Other Resources appendix of this book.

Helping Other People

After struggling through the uncertainties of cancer treatment, many people find that participating in a self-help group for cancer survivors is quite rewarding. Having found the courage or the endurance to face down cancer, you have valuable experience and knowledge you can share with another person. The experience of sharing can enrich your life, give your self-esteem a lift, and benefit another person. One such program is the American Cancer Society's CanSurmount program, which connects people who have been cured of cancer with newly diagnosed cancer patients.

People find their own ways to contribute. One entrepreneur who recovered from leukemia started his own private golf tournament, which has already raised thousands of dollars for the American Leukemia Society.

On a spiritual, psychological, and even social level, many people have found that facing their own mortality has given new meaning to their lives. Some people claim to have a new focus on the essentials of life and a new ability to ignore trivial problems. A few people who have been unhappy and disappointed with their lives before being diagnosed with cancer have discovered a reservoir of joy they didn't realize they had inside them.

You may find your life changed after your cancer is in remission, but these changes are manageable. Go back for medical checkups as recommended. Work to communicate your feelings to people around you and to hear what your friends and family members have to say. Know that discrimination at work can occur, but that legal remedies are available. Perhaps most importantly, try to maintain a healthy lifestyle after recovering from cancer, because living a healthy life will lessen your chances for a recurrence.

Unfortunately, sometimes chemotherapy doesn't work—the subject of the following chapter.

21

WHEN CHEMOTHERAPY DOESN'T WORK

FACING MORE CHEMOTHERAPY OR FACING YOUR OWN MORTALITY

THIS CHAPTER DEALS WITH ISSUES THAT ARISE WHEN CHEMOTHERAPY either doesn't work or isn't effective. Questions about additional treatment will arise, and suggestions are included for making this process easier. You may want to consider a hospice program, which can provide a safe and comfortable place for a person to spend their last days. If your cancer is terminal, preparations can be made to make the experience easier on survivors and ease your peace of mind.

Sometimes the first round of chemotherapy simply doesn't work. At this point, if the doctor recommends it, you must decide whether to undergo "second stage" chemotherapy with different drugs, or even try a "third stage" chemotherapy treatment after that. This is an extremely difficult decision for both patient and doctor, because the chances of a response are less the second and third times around although a positive response is still possible. Your own philosophy regarding treatment, and the philosophy of your doctor, will factor into this decision.

As in the beginning, a second medical opinion can be useful. You may consider entering a clinical trial, the benefits of which are discussed in this book in chapter 6, especially if you can find one that offers some real chance of success in treating your cancer. If you enter into more medical treatment, you will need to have a very frank discussion with your oncologist about the risks and benefits of undergoing further chemotherapy.

At some point, you may find yourself in the position of having a type of cancer that cannot be controlled by current medical practice. At that point, you may just want to consider the possibility of living out your life in circumstances that are as comfortable and enjoyable to you as possible. Research psychologist Lawrence LeShahn has written of some remarkable successes with terminally ill cancer patients. LeShahn's books relate the tales of a few terminally ill patients who made remarkable and sustained recoveries for long periods of time after they discovered and pursued their real interests in life.

Dr. Bernie Siegel tells the story of a young lawyer who had always wanted to be a violinist, but who felt forced by his parents to succeed in the legal profession. The young lawyer developed a tumor in his brain, and was given a year to live by his doctors. When he heard the news he reportedly stated, "Then I will play my violin for a year." A year later, the former lawyer was playing violin in an orchestra and his brain tumor had vanished.

"When we die and we go to heaven, and we meet our Maker, our Maker is not going to say to us, why didn't you become a messiah? Why didn't you discover the cure for such and such? The only thing we're going to be asked at that precious moment is why didn't you become *you*?" writes Eli Wiesel in his book, *Souls on Fire.*

Human Mortality

Accepting one's own mortality, or perhaps even the possibility of one's mortality, involves a series of five psychological plateaus first delineated by author Elisabeth Kübler-Ross—denial, anger, bargaining or guilt, depression, and, finally, acceptance.

You may go through all these stages after you are diagnosed with cancer, and possibly at key points during your illness. Crisis points at which you may expect to experience the most emotional stress include the end of chemotherapy treatment, upon learning of the failure of conventional treatment, when you have a recurrence of cancer, and when you begin an investigational treatment. The strongest experience of all may come if you learn that your cancer is terminal.

Your family and your friends may experience strong emotional reactions, too. Sometimes families draw closer together in such situations, and friendships become permanent. But some people withdraw, because they don't have the faintest idea of what to say or how to say it. Remember that some of the greatest words of solace have always been, "I love you, regardless and always."

At this critical juncture, nearly overwhelming fears may roll over you like waves, for a long time. The fear of the unknown, the fear of being abandoned, the fear of becoming a burden, the fear of leaving unfinished business, and the fear for the future of your loved ones are all commonly felt by people who are seriously ill. You might get depressed for what seems like an eternity, or angry at yourself. According to Kübler-Ross, another constant in all five stages is hope. Hope helps people literally fight for their life and hold onto themselves through long periods of physical suffering.

If you feel completely overwhelmed by the circumstances of your life, consider entering a support group. Seek individual or group counseling from a psychotherapist or a religious counselor affiliated with your church, synagogue, or mosque. Chaplains and psychologists are available in most hospitals, and they will see you any time you request to see them. Using the stress-relieving techniques listed in chapter 16 will help you maintain the quality of your life, help you manage pain, and make your own death more comfortable.

If you're a spiritual person, you may be interested in research published in 1988, which turned up what appears to be scientific proof of the healing power of prayer. At the University of California at San Francisco, Randy Byrd, a cardiologist, did a double-blind study of patients who had experienced heart problems. The group was randomly divided in half, and half the patients were prayed for and half were not prayed for. The patients who were prayed for had less incidence of pulmonary edema, needed less intubation, and needed less antibiotics than the control group.

Still, religious doubt can develop in any serious sickness, and even some very religious people go through a long period of feeling that God has deserted them. Religious doubts during cancer treatment are said to most frequently appear in patients who have an idea of a benevolent Higher Power who rewards the faithful and punishes the faithless. Prayer remains extraordinarily comforting to many people because they feel it connects them with something much larger and more permanent than themselves.

Serenity Prayer

The *Serenity Prayer*, written by theologian Reinhold Niebuhr, is a useful tool for some people because it helps them sort through and prioritize their personal experiences. A short version of the *Serenity Prayer* used by many Twelve Step programs goes:

> God grant me the serenity
> To accept the things I cannot change,
> The courage to change the things I can,
> And the wisdom to know the difference.

This short prayer can be extraordinarily comforting, which is probably why it is called the *Serenity Prayer.* Just saying this short prayer aloud or to yourself when you feel stressed may actually help you feel more serene.

And of course, religion may just not be for you. Although a few nonbelievers do have a religious experience on their deathbed, a lot of research shows that most people die about the same way they lived, that is, they hold onto the values that have sustained them in life even when they know they are dying.

There is no question that approaching death is a profoundly lonely and frightening concept to face. We all know we are mortal, but we don't expect to literally watch and feel ourselves decline. The psychiatrist Thomas P. Hackett has observed, "Those who are going to die fear the process of dying more than death itself."

Medication

Unfortunately, a tendency exists for terminal patients to be over-medicated in the last days of their lives, perhaps itself a reaction by physicians to the idea that medicine should be able to cure everything. It is interesting to note that physicians express the failures of medical treatment among themselves by saying, "The patient didn't respond to the treatment." This way of expressing the failure of medical treatment puts the onus of responding to cancer treatment on the patient rather than the physician. The terminology alone indicates a subliminal wish to believe that dying is somehow the patient's fault, or at least not the fault of the physician, who presumably did his or her best to rid the patient of disease and was powerful enough to do so.

Physicians are quite human. Some may unconsciously feel that a dying patient is a personal failure, and not wish to face the unanswerable questions that a terminal patient may ask. Like doctors, nurses and other health-care workers receive gratification through healing and may unconsciously avoid the terminally ill patient because they fear discussing their death. Terminally ill and elderly patients do have a right to relief from pain. But pain relief is different from being tranquilized into an unnecessary haze of speechlessness during your final days.

Despite the work of Kübler-Ross and others in the field, talking about death remains taboo in American society. We tend to bottle up these feelings and not discuss them. Some of the largest cancer centers have memorial services for their patients among the staff, and even pay the staff to attend them, because the best treatment facilities are beginning to realize that it's important for people who work with the seriously ill to work through the feelings they may have about death to avoid burning out in their jobs.

The fact remains that cancer is an extraordinarily powerful and complex set of diseases, for which modern medical science has no "magic bullet" vaccine, or even a guaranteed cure. Sometimes the biology of cancer simply overwhelms the human body, and the disease overwhelms the best efforts made by either the doctor, the support team, or even medical science itself.

Home Care

Most certainly, most of us would prefer to spend our last months at home, in the company of people we know, rather than in an institutional setting. This is sometimes possible, depending on the medical condition of the patient and financial and other circumstances. Visiting nurses can be utilized. Your medical team is a good source of referrals for experienced home care nurses. If family members attempt to take the patient home, the family must be up to the very demanding task of caring for the person with cancer. Of course, financial and other considerations will factor into this decision.

One social worker tells the story of a family whose young daughter was terminally ill and in the hospital. The girl was given only a few days to live by her doctors. Home care was expensive, but it was available, and since the doctors only expected it to be a matter of days before the daughter died, the social worker urged the girl's family to take her home from the hospital. The girl lived for many, many weeks longer than expected, and the costs of home care mounted much higher than had been anticipated—imposing a substantial financial burden on the parents. The social worker felt guilty, the parents were left with enormous bills, but the girl died at home.

This example shows that doctors have no completely accurate way of predicting any person's life span, since the rate at which a particular cancer progresses is difficult to predict accurately. Home care planning should certainly involve financial planning. To the parents of this child, it may have still been worthwhile to have the girl at home for her final weeks despite the enormous expense.

Many hospitals and community institutions have begun to help cancer patients and their families cope with the difficulties of caring for a very ill patient. Some of these programs are called "home oncology medical extension programs," or sometimes they are called hospice programs.

Hospices

The hospice concept was begun in England by Cicely Saunders, M.D. In 1967 Dr. Saunders founded St. Christopher's Hospice as a place for terminally ill patients and their families to receive practical support and help, rather than continued medical treatment if that was no longer of value to the patient. St. Christopher's was so obviously of comfort and value to its patients that it sparked the hospice movement, which has revolutionized thinking on how to care for the terminally ill.

The hospice movement has the great virtue of aiming to make the patient as comfortable as possible during his or her last days, in a nonhospital setting. The vitality and growth of the hospice movement itself is a statement that maintaining the highest possible quality of life until the end of life is important.

Today in the United States, hospices can be stand-alone facilities in separate locations, or located within a hospital or nursing facility. Many involve home care programs radiating out from a particular hospital—which is quite convenient, since patients may be taken back and forth to a particular hospital for medical treatment. In addition to terminal cancer patients, both adults and children, hospices now exist for people with other conditions that limit their life expectancy such as AIDS and Alzheimer's disease.

Frequently run by religious organizations, many hospices offer spiritual and emotional counseling. Hospice personnel aim to make the patient as comfortable as possible physically and mentally, but use no "heroic" measures to prolong life. Some also offer respite services to family members caring for a sick relative, during which they will temporarily take over the care of a patient to give family members a chance to rest and relax.

Under current United States law, always subject to revision, cancer patients who are covered by Medicare and not expected to live more than six months who need treatment for the symptoms

233

of cancer, or control of pain, are entitled to 210 days of home care through hospice programs. Check with Social Security Administration offices, hospices, home health care agencies, visiting nurse associations, or hospital social service departments for the latest rules on this.

In this age of financial constraints, it's interesting to note that hospice care is the only new treatment approved by Medicare in recent years. Its approval under Medicare Part A, which is the hospital insurance care portion of our national health insurance program for senior citizens, is a testament both to the success of the hospice as a humane treatment and as one that is also more cost-effective than a hospital stay. Hospice referrals may be found in the Other Resources appendix of this book.

Planning for Death

Many, many survivors are not prepared to handle the responsibilities and immediate needs that occur when a loved one dies. Up to 90 percent of survivors are unprepared, according to one estimate. Planning for your death is an expression of how you wish your affairs handled. Planning can make your death less difficult for those left behind.

In many states, if you can no longer make decisions about your medical treatment, your doctor will ask your closest available relative or friend to help decide a course of action. If you have strong feelings about who should make medical decisions for you, you can legally give that person power of attorney for your health care and provide copies of the form you sign to both your doctor and the person to whom you give this authority. If you don't want any heroic and expensive medical treatment to prolong your life past a certain point, have a living will or declaration drawn up that states your wishes.

One book, *Legacy of Love* by Elmo A. Petterle, helps you start planning for your death by preparing a will. Among other things, this book covers how you wish to be cared for if you become seriously ill, and includes instructions for making a living will and durable powers of attorney. It also asks for your choice of cemetery or mortuary, the type of funeral service or memorial service you wish, and provides advice on death benefits available in the United States. It asks you to list your assets, including home, health, and casualty insurance. It asks for medical history information of potential use to your descendants. Most importantly, it requests that you provide your survivors with a list of telephone numbers for people you may wish notified of your demise such as the post office or clubs, organizations, or church groups. Collecting this information in advance will help your survivors get through their own period of mourning with a minimum of trouble and give them an idea of how you might wish them to proceed.

Another book, *The Diagnosis Is Cancer* by Edward J. Larschan, J.D., Ph.D., and Richard Larschan, Ph.D., spells out the legal arrangements and other practical matters that survivors will need to know.

NEW TREATMENTS

No ONE REALLY KNOWS WHERE THE NEXT BREAKTHROUGHS IN CANCER treatment will appear. At this moment, thousands of research projects are underway all over the United States, and indeed all over the world. Promising new areas of treatment are currently the subject of a lot of research, and may someday be of wide benefit. They include:

Biological Therapy

Immunotherapy is in its infancy and still primarily investigational, but is an accepted treatment for a few types of cancer. For instance, interferon-alpha is an approved treatment for hairy cell leukemia and Kaposi's sarcoma. Generally speaking, biological therapy is genetic engineering, which aims to stimulate the immune system with purified proteins such as interferon and interleukin-2, and to activate the body's natural defenses to fight cancer cells. Colony-stimulating factors, T cells, and tumor necrosis factors are also being studied for their antitumor effects. Antibody therapy involving monoclonal antibodies, which search out and destroy cancer cells, and other antibodies made in the laboratory also shows promise. Monoclonal antibodies are currently being used to remove cancer cells from stored bone marrow, before it's transplanted back into the patient, but antigens in cancer cells can develop something like resistance to monoclonal antibodies. Experimental work is also underway with monoclonal antibodies being attached to chemotherapy drugs by chemical bonding, allowing the therapy to bring the chemotherapy drugs directly to the tumor cells and not to the rest of the body, thereby decreasing the toxic side effects of the drugs to normal noncancerous cells.

Gene Therapy

Attempts are being made to "package and deliver" genetic information to cells at the molecular level. Although it is a difficult process, scientists are working to insert genes into "stem" or progenitor cells, and to vector genes on target cells to treat blood and immunologic disorders. This research could benefit the four thousand disorders that are known to have genetic roots, including cancer, heart disease, arthritis, and AIDS. For instance, the MDR1 gene has already been identified as a gene that resists chemotherapy drugs.

Another aspect of gene therapy is the "lock and key" approach, which aims to develop drugs that block certain proteins controlling the chemical codes within human DNA, and thereby "locking off" the genes that control the division of cancer cells. For instance, a couple of experimental new chemical compounds show some capacity to block the *ras* oncogene, a gene that can make cells cancerous—in effect "switching off" the growth of about 20 percent of human cancers believed linked to this oncogene. This research has the potential to create a new type of chemotherapy with a much more specific action than most chemotherapy drugs now in use and no side effects.

The Human Genome Project is a multibillion-dollar research effort that will "map" each of the human body's 100,000 genes and help contribute to our understanding of the role of genes in the formation of both normal and cancerous cells in humans.

Bone Marrow Transplantation

Since the bone marrow is the organ of the body most sensitive to chemotherapy drugs and radiation, bone marrow transplantation is sometimes used as a way to allow more powerful doses of anticancer drugs to be used to fight cancer. Normal bone marrow is withdrawn for protection prior to administration of chemotherapy, and then reinfused after chemotherapy is finished. Increases in doses of chemotherapy drugs of up to 500 percent are possible, making the difference in some cases between the palliation and cure of cancer. Bone marrow transplantation is an expensive and dangerous treatment, but useful for patients who can be cured with higher doses of chemotherapy than the bone marrow would normally allow.

Chemoprevention

The greatest reductions in cancer rates may well come from prevention. The American Cancer Society's emphasis on a more low-fat, high-fiber diet is the result of many studies that show such diets result in lower rates of cancer. Several dozen research studies involving vitamin A, vitamin C, and other vitamins and minerals are now underway to test dietary and other preventative strategies—which may eventually teach us how to live a lifestyle that prevents both initial cases and recurrences of cancer.

Psychoneuroimmunology

This long term is a formal scientific name for the interaction of the mind and the emotions on the immune system. Research indicates that the immune system is enhanced by positive emotions such as laughter and may be weakened by long-term unpleasant emotions. It is theorized that a strong immune system may help the body recover from illness, and that discoveries in this area may have some effect on the prevention and the treatment of a disease such as cancer.

OTHER RESOURCES

MANY FINE RESOURCES EXIST TO HELP THE PERSON WITH CANCER and their families. The following organizations can provide useful information, and in some cases even financial or practical assistance. This is only a partial list of the organizations that exist, but contacting a few of the larger organizations can help put you in touch with many others. A selected listing of electronic databases and electronic addresses, plus a reading list of recommended books on cancer and chemotherapy, are also included here.

National Cancer Institute (NCI)

The National Cancer Institute is a division of the National Institutes of Health, which are all under the U.S. Department of Health and Human Services.

The NCI is a primary source for medical information about cancer, including information on particular anticancer drugs, medical facilities, physician referrals, second opinion centers, and investigational trials. Information is distributed free of charge through the Cancer Information Service (CIS). A number of excellent publications are available on topics such as chemotherapy, diet, and coping with family issues. This valuable information service for cancer patients and their families may be reached toll-free. Spanish-speaking operators are available in the United States.

In Canada, the Ontario Cancer Information Service distributes similar factual material to Canadians.

The Physicians' Data Query (PDQ) computer database may also be found at the NCI's toll-free number. PDQ includes free state-of-the-art treatment information, information on chemotherapy drugs, information about current clinical trials, data on other organizations, and credentials information on doctors involved in caring for people who have cancer. Your doctor may access this database to find out the latest and best treatments for your type of cancer. Also, a new "patient's version" of clinical trial information is available, which may be provided to your doctor. CancerFax provides a way to receive PDQ information statements in English or Spanish via fax. CancerNet serves the same function utilizing electronic mail. Both CancerFax and CancerNet are free services provided by the federal government.

National Cancer Institute, Building 31, Room 1024A, Bethesda, MD 20892. Telephone (800) 422-6237.

Ontario Cancer Information Service, 755 Concession Street, Hamilton, Ontario L8V 1C4. Telephone (800) 263-6750 inside Canada; or (905) 387-0376.

American Cancer Society (ACS)

The American Cancer Society is a large private organization that raises funds and provides a number of support services for cancer patients. The Canadian Cancer Society is a similar organization located in Canada. The ACS is active in a great many areas, including treatment options and prevention. The ACS provides a number of free informational booklets about cancer. Local ACS chapters often have "loan chest" program which loan items such as wigs, wheelchairs, and other cancer-related supplies to people who need them. The ACS provides referrals for second medical opinions and a number of support services. Local offices of the ACS may also provide information on "wish fulfillment" programs for children with cancer. The ACS has a home page on the Internet, and an electronic address on America Online.

American Cancer Society National Office, 1599 Clifton

Road, NE, Atlanta, GA 30329. Telephone (800) ACS-2345; (800) 227-2345.

Canadian Cancer Society, 10 Alcorn Avenue, Suite 200, Toronto, Ontario M4V3B1. Telephone (416) 961-7223.

Financial Aid

A listing of drug manufacturers' hot line services is available on request from the **Association of Community Cancer Centers** (ACCC), 11600 Nebel Street, #201, Rockville, MD 20852; telephone (301) 984-9496. When contacted, manufacturers' hot lines will often provide free drugs to needy patients. These hot lines also may assist you to get reimbursed by your insurance company if payment reimbursement is denied for one of their company's chemotherapy drugs.

The **NCI** also provides drug manufacturers' hot line numbers at (800) 422-6237.

The Leukemia Society of America, 800 Second Avenue, New York, NY 10017, provides some financial assistance for out-patient care and referrals to other potential sources of help for people with leukemia. Telephone (800) 955-4572.

The Pediatric Branch, National Cancer Institute, National Institutes of Health, Building 10, Room 13 N 240, Bethesda, MD 20892, offers free medical treatment and related services for several hundred pediatric cancer patients each year as well as informational publications. Telephone (301) 496-4256.

American Cancer Society, National Office, 1599 Clifton Road, NE, Atlanta, GA 30329. Telephone (800) ACS-2345; (800) 227-2345.

Canadian Cancer Society, 10 Alcorn Avenue, Suite 200, Toronto, Ontario M4V 3B1. Telephone (416) 961-7223.

Support Groups and Support Services

The American Cancer Society sponsors a number of support programs including the "I Can Cope" program for cancer patients and their families, the "CanSurmount" program for newly-diagnosed cancer patients, and the "Reach for Recovery" program for breast cancer patients at (800) ACS-2345.

The National Cancer Foundation, 1180 Avenue of the Americas, New York, NY 10036, promotes social services for cancer patients, including free counseling and group therapy. Telephone (212) 221-3300.

Make Today Count, P.O. Box 303, Burlington, IA 52601. Telephone (319) 753-6521.

Y-ME Breast Cancer Support Program, 212 W. Van Buren Street, 4th Floor, Chicago, IL 60607. Telephone (800) 221-2141.

US-Too, International, prostate cancer support, 930 N. York Road #50, Hinsdale, IL 60521-2993. Telephone (800) 808-7866.

Wellness Community, 1235 5th Street, Santa Monica, CA 90401. Telephone (800) PRO-HOPE.

Cancervive, 6500 Wilshire Boulevard, #500, Los Angeles, CA 90048. Telephone (310) 203-9232.

Visiting Nurse Assn. of America, 3801 E. Florida Ave., #900, Denver, Co 80210. Telephone (800) 426-2547.

Biofeedback

To find a clinical person skilled in biofeedback contact the **Association for Applied Psychophysiology and Biofeedback,** 10200 W. 44th Avenue, #304, Wheat Ridge, CO 80033. Telephone (300) 477-8892.

Hypnosis

Referrals to state organizations of clinicians who are skilled in treating illness with hypnosis through the **American Society of Clinical Hypnosis,** 2200 E. Devon Avenue, #291, Des Plaines, IL 60018-4534. Telephone (708) 297-3317.

Visual Imaging

The Simonton Cancer Center, P.O. Box 890, Pacific Palisades, CA 90272, can refer to physicians, nurses, or psychologists who have gone through their visual imaging training program.

Telephone (800) 459-3424; tapes (800) 338-2360; administration (310) 457-3811.

Air Transportation

The Corporate Angel Network, Westchester County Airport, White Plains, NY 10604, provides free transportation all across the United States for ambulatory cancer patients who have medical authorization for the travel to treatment centers on corporate aircraft. Telephone (914) 328-1313.

Pediatric Cancer

The Candlelighters Childhood Cancer Foundation, 7910 Woodmont Avenue, Bethesda, MD 20814, provides support, education and advocacy programs for families of children with cancer. Telephone (800) 366-2223.

The National Children's Cancer Society, Inc., 1015 Locust Building, #1040, St. Louis, MO 63101, offers financial assistance for children who need a bone marrow transplant. Telephone (800) 882-NCCS.

Ronald McDonald Houses, One Kroc Drive, Oak Brook, IL 60521, provide lodging for families of pediatric cancer patients near some pediatric hospitals for a small fee. Telephone (708) 575-7048.

Children's Hospice International, Suite 700, 700 Princess Street, Lower Level, Alexandria, VA 22314, is a network of support for terminally ill children and their families. Telephone (800) 242-4453.

Amie Karen Cancer Fund for Children, P.O. Box 17926, Beverly Hills, CA 90209. Telephone (310) 335-5330.

Insurance/Job Discrimination

The National Coalition for Cancer Survivorship (NCCS), 1010 Wayne Avenue, 5th Floor, Silver Spring, MD 20910, is a cancer patient advocacy organization composed of individuals and groups with information on insurance, community support groups, and employment discrimination as it affects cancer survivors. The *NCCS Networker* newsletter lists other newsletters that deal with specific cancers, such as breast cancer or prostate cancer. Telephone (301) 650-8868.

The insurance industry sponsors the **National Consumer Insurance Helpline** (800) 942-4242.

The Medicare Information Line provides information on Medicare, Medicare supplemental insurance, Medicare claims, mammograms, HMOs, and special programs for low income people at (800) 638-6833.

U.S. Equal Employment Opportunity Commission (800) 872-3362.

National Rehabilitation Information Center (800) 34-NARIC.

Pain Management

The American Pain Society will provide a listing of pain clinics and specialized treatment centers. Telephone (708) 966-5595.

Look Good, Feel Better

The **"Look Good . . . Feel Better"** program is a free educational program for individuals undergoing chemotherapy or radiation therapy that offers tips on restoring your appearance during treatments. Sessions are usually in small groups. Telephone (800) 395-LOOK.

Oncology Referrals

To locate a board-certified medical oncologist in your area or to check the professional credentials of an oncologist, contact the **American Society of Clinical Oncology,** 435 N. Michigan Avenue, #1717, Chicago, IL 60611. Telephone (312) 644-0828.

Unorthodox Cancer Treatments

The National Council Against Health Fraud, P.O. Box 1276, Loma Linda, CA 92354, collects information and publishes position papers on unproven cancer cures. Telephone (909) 824-4690.

Chemotherapy

The Chemotherapy Foundation, Inc., 183 Madison Avenue, New York, NY 10016, conducts research and offers pamphlets on chemotherapy, breast cancer, and ovarian cancer. Telephone (212) 213-9292.

Sex Therapy

The American Association of Sex Educators, Counselors, and Therapists, 435 North Michigan Avenue, #1717, Chicago, IL 60611, is the principal professional organization in the sexual therapy field, and can refer you to a practitioner in your area. Telephone (312) 644-0828.

Ostomies

The United Ostomy Association, 36 Executive Park, #120, Irvine, CA 92714. Provides information, including data on support groups. Telephone (800) 826-0826.

Hospices

The National Hospice Organization in Arlington, VA, can provide names and addresses of hospices in your area. Telephone (800) 658-8898.

The Hospice Education Institute offers referrals to local hospices at (800) 331-1620.

Computer Databases

CANCERLIT is a database of the National Library of Medicine in Betheseda, MD. Contains journal articles, books, and other information on all aspects of cancer research and treatment including abstracts for many, and clinical trial information. Cancerlit is available for a fee through interfaces such as Colleague, itself available from companies such as Ovid Technologies. Telephone (800) 950-2035.

MEDLARS, MEDLINE, and other computerized databases, available at many college and medical libraries, contain listings of published articles and books on medical topics.

Information on several National Library of Medicine programs and services is available at (800) 272-4787.

Internet Addresses

sci.med
sci.bio
These are discussion forums for medical and scientific professionals, students, and people curious about these issues.

alt.support.cancer
sci.med.diseases.cancer
On-line discussion groups.

cancer.med.upenn.edu 80
University of Pennsylvania's OncoLink.

cancernetaicicc.nci.nih.gov
National Cancer Institute.

World Wide Web Home Pages

http://wwwicic,NCI.NIH.GOV/
On-line information from the National Cancer Institute.

http://www.cancer.org/
American Cancer Society information.

http://www.nlm.nih.gov/
National Library of Medicine.

http://vh.radiology.uIowa.edu/
The University of Iowa's "Virtual Hospital"—includes such things as multimedia medical textbooks, patient simulations, and computer gateways to other medical resources.

http://cancer.med.upenn.edu/
The University of Pennsylvania's Oncolink.

http://hyrax.med.uth.tmc.edu/
The University of Texas on-line center for medical information.

http://access.digex.net/∼mkragen/cansearch.htm/
NCCS guide to on-line resources.

Other Reading

Benjamin, Harold. *From Victim to Victor.* Los Angeles: J.P. Tarcher, 1987.

Bracken, Jeanne Munn. *Children with Cancer: A Comprehensive Reference Guide for Parents.* New York: Oxford University Press, 1986.

Bruning, Nancy. *Coping with Chemotherapy: How to Take Care of Yourself While Chemotherapy Takes Care of the Cancer.* Garden City: Dial Press, 1985.

Cousins, Norman. *Anatomy of an Illness as Perceived by the Patient: Reflections on Healing and Regeneration.* New York: W.W. Norton & Co., 1979.

Dollinger, Malin, M.D., Rosenbaum, Ernest H., M.D., and Cable, Greg. *Everyone's Guide to Cancer Therapy: How Cancer Is Diagnosed, Treated and Managed Day to Day.* Toronto: Somerville House Books Ltd., 1991.

Harpham, Wendy Schlessel, M.D. *Diagnosis Cancer: Your Guide Through the First Few Months.* New York: W.W. Norton & Co., 1992.

Lindsay, Anne. *The American Cancer Society Cookbook.* New York: William Morrow & Co., 1988.

Reich, Paul R., M.D., with Janice E. Metcalf. *The Facts about Chemotherapy: The Essential Guide for Cancer Patients and Their Families*. Mount Vernon: Consumer Reports Books, 1991.

Siegel, Bernie. *Love, Medicine and Miracles*. New York: Harper Collins, 1986.

Simonton, Carl O., and Stephanie Matthews-Simonton. *Getting Well Again*. Los Angeles: J.P. Tarcher, 1978.

APPENDIX

GLOSSARY OF COMMON TERMS

Adjuvant chemotherapy   Chemotherapy given as a preventative measure after surgery or radiation treatments have removed a cancer. Given to rid the body of any leftover cancer that may be undetectable.

Alopecia   A medical term for the complete or partial loss of hair.

Alkylating agents   A family of anticancer drugs that prevent division in the cancer cell.

Anemia   A condition caused by having too few red blood cells, which results in a tired, breathless, physically weak feeling.

Anorexia   A medical term for poor appetite.

Antiemetic   A medicine that helps control vomiting.

Antimetabolites   A family of anticancer drugs that act by fooling cancer cells into thinking they are vitamins that will nourish cancer cell growth.

Benign tumor   A growth that is not cancerous.

Biological response modifiers   Substances that either occur in nature or are man-made that can modify the response of the immune system, and help fight and control cancer.

Biopsy   A medical procedure to remove a piece of tissue to examine it under a microscope.

Blood count   A complete blood count (CBC) is a test that calculates the number of red blood cells, white blood cells, and platelets in your body. The CBC is useful in determining the effects of chemotherapy on a particular patient.

Bone marrow   Inner tissue of larger bones where red blood cells and white blood cells are made.

Cancer   A group of more than two-hundred diseases characterized by abnormal cell growth. Also a name for a malignant tumor.

Catheter   A plastic tube inserted into the body to inject fluids into the body, or to withdraw bodily fluids.

Chemotherapy   The treatment of cancer with chemicals designed to stop the growth or spread of cancer.

Clinical trials   Controlled scientific tests involving human beings that compare new methods of cancer treatment against older methods.

CT or CAT scan   A computed axial tomography scan is an x-ray procedure that shows cross sections of the body.

Combination chemotherapy   The use of more than one drug at a time to treat cancer.

Cure   In cancer treatment, normally this means that a person has about the same life expectancy as if they hadn't had cancer. Often, the term is used when the cancer has been in remission for at least five years.

Diagnosis   The process by which a doctor identifies the nature of a disease, prior to treating it.

Gastrointestinal   A medical term for the digestive tract, which includes the mouth, esophagus, stomach, and intestines.

Hormones   Substances released by one organ in the body that can affect the function of other organs.

Hormonal therapy   The therapeutic administration of hormones to block the action of other hormones to slow the growth of cancer.

Hospice   A place where terminally ill patients receive care to keep them as comfortable as possible during their last days of life.

Immune system   The natural mechanisms that your body uses to ward off germs and disease.

Immunotherapy Stimulating the body's immune defense systems to treat or help treat a medical condition such as cancer.

Informed consent The legal standard that states that a patient must know certain risks and benefits regarding therapy before agreeing to take it.

Infusion Intravenous delivery of a chemotherapy drug or fluids made in a slow or prolonged manner.

Injection A shot.

Lesion A mass of cells.

Localized A cancer that is limited to the site at which it originated, with no evidence that the cancer has spread.

Lymphatic system Our body's thousands of lymph nodes comprise a lymph system containing a clear fluid that carries white blood cells that combat infection to various parts of the body.

Malignant tumor A cancerous growth.

Metastasis The spread of cancer from its original location to another location in the body.

National Cancer Institute The prestigious national research center located in Bethesda, Maryland, which supervises clinical trials for new cancer treatments all across the United States and also provides information to the public regarding many aspects of the treatment of cancer.

Nodule A small mass of tissue, frequently malignant.

Oncologist A doctor who specializes in cancer treatment. Medical oncologists treat cancer with chemotherapy. Radiation oncologists treat cancer with radiation therapy. Surgical oncologists treat cancer with surgery.

Palliation Treatment given to arrest cancer, rather than to eradicate the disease, given for a purpose such as arresting pain.

Primary tumor The tumor where cancer originates, which "names" the cancer, regardless of where it spreads. If your cancer originates in your lungs, for instance, your primary tumor is lung cancer. Also called the primary site.

Prognosis A medical prediction of how a patient will do in the future, based on statistics and the physician's evaluation of a particular patient.

Protocol The steps of a particular medical treatment or procedure, given in a particular sequence, which are written down.

Radiation therapy The treatment of cancer with high-energy rays.

Recurrence The reappearance of cancer after a period of apparent remission.

Regression A shrinking of a tumor, or slowing of cancer growth.

Remission A partial or a complete shrinkage of a cancer due to chemotherapy or other treatment.

Side effects Symptoms that relate directly to medical treatment, such as nausea after a chemotherapy treatment. Side effects are either *acute,* meaning that they occur during treatment, or *chronic,* meaning that their effects can linger for a period of time.

Staging Evaluation of cancer to see the extent to which it has grown or spread in relation to the normal progress of the disease.

Stomatitis Medical term for sores found on the inside lining of the mouth.

Suppository A way of administering medicines that involves insertion through the rectum or vagina.

Support group A group of people who have cancer or whose cancer is in remission who meet periodically to exchange information and discuss medical treatment and life issues. Support groups may also focus on or include spouses and families of cancer patients.

Supportive care services Dr. Paul Coluzzi defines supportive care services as "those medical and psychosocial services that promote and enhance the quality of life for patients with cancer through education, research, and clinical service." Provided in a hospital setting, support services can include such things as psychotherapy, support groups, hypnosis, pain clinics, and even pet therapy.

Systemic   Something such as a chemotherapy treatment that affects the whole body rather than just one part of it.

Toxic reaction   Side effects or reactions to poisons that are potentially quite serious.

Tumor   An abnormal mass of tissue that may be either benign (noncancerous) or malignant (cancerous).

Tumor markers   Tests that indicate the status of a tumor.

X-rays   Electromagnetic radiation that passes through the body to provide an image of the inside of the body on film.

INDEX

death of cancer cells, 27
death, planning for, 234–235
dehydration, 115, 119, 120, 126, 127,
  139–140, 154
denial of insurance coverage, 207
Department of Agriculture (USDA),
  148–149
Department of Health, 50
depression, 35, 118, 129, 136, 142, 158,
  162, 167, 171–178, 188
dental care, 65, 114, 123, 128–129
designated person, 70
Diagnosis Cancer, 249
Diagnosis Is Cancer, 235
diarrhea, 114, 124–125, 139, 143
diary, benefits of keeping, 90
diet as risk factor for cancer, 144–148
dietary control of
  constipation, 125–126
  diarrhea, 139
  fatigue, 120
  fluid retention, 128
  infection, 121
  kidney and bladder problems,
    127–128
  loss of appetite, 119
  mouth and throat problems,
    123–124
  nausea, 115
dieticians, 68, 139, 150
Dilaudid, 162
disability insurance, 208
discrimination at work, 224–225,
  245–246
distraction, 77, 160, 179, 183–184
Divine Comedy, 174
dizziness, 120
DNA effects, 25, 94
doctors' arrogance, 64
doctors' expertise, 64, 143, 246
Dollinger, Malin, M.D., 91, 249
Donnatel, 124
doubling of cancer cells, 16, 25
doxorubicin (Adriamycin), 26, 73, 94,
  100–101, 140, 201
drug addiction, 163–164
drug companies, help from, 205–206

drug dependence, 163
dry mouth, tips to relieve, 119

easy-to-eat foods, 124
education, value for patients, 9, 23, 31,
  34, 65, 81–92, 93, 160, 183, 192
efficacy trials, 60
Ekman, Paul, M.D., 167
Ellington, Duke, 4
emotional aspects, xvi, xvii, 3, 9, 14, 35,
  51, 52, 58, 65, 129–130, 151–155,
  165–178, 221–222, 228–229
emotional stress, effects and relief,
  129–130, 136, 165–178, 228–229
emotional support, 187–197, 221–222,
  228–229
endometrium, 99, 100, 107, 145
Ensure, 119, 124
enzymes, 94
Equal Opportunity Commission, 246
Erickson, Milton, 181
erythropoietin, 72
esophagus, cancer of the, 105, 145
estradiol (Estraderm), 101
estramustine (Emcyt), 101, 201
estrogens, 43–44, 101–102
etoposide (VePesid et al.), 20, 103, 114,
  201
Everyone's Guide to Cancer Therapy, 91,
  223, 249
"exceptional patients," 167
exercise, benefits of, 68, 125, 138, 141,
  143, 148, 152, 160, 179, 183–185,
  223, 224
experimental treatments, 41, 42, 59–61,
  202, 209, 227–228, 237–239
expertise of specialists, 67–68
eyes, precautions to take, 153

Facts about Chemotherapy, 249
failure of treatment, 227–235
false menopause, 129
family issues, 21,49, 51, 70, 72–73, 141,
  169–170, 173, 175–178, 187–190,
  192, 193, 196, 221, 229, 232
famous people with cancer, 4, 212
fasting, danger of, 115

Index

LeShahn, Lawrence, 188, 228
lesions, 253
leucovorin (folinic acid et al.), 26, 104, 201
leukemia, 15, 17, 26, 51, 86–89, 94, 97, 98, 99, 100, 102, 103, 105, 106, 108, 109, 166, 237, 243
Leukemia Society of America, 209, 243
leuprolide (Lupron et al.), 104, 201
levamisole (Ergamisol), 26, 104
library, use of, 91, 247–248
life-saving treatments, 202
life span of cancer patients; *also see* statistics
life support systems, 40, 233
Lindsay, Anne, 249
liquid diet, 125
liver cancer, 102
liver, effects on, 138
liver scans, 38
living will, 41, 210
"loan chest" programs, 117, 242
local treatment, advantages of, 62
localized cancer, definition, 253
"lock and key" approach, 238
Lomotil, 124
lomustine (CCNU et al.), 104, 140, 201
"Look Good, Feel Better" program, 152, 246
loss of appetite, 113, 118–119, 136–137, 141–142, 149
loss of balance, 126
loss of control, 23, 36, 136, 161, 174, 213
loss of hair, *see* hair loss; wigs and hairpieces
loss of weight, 30, 136–137, 149–150, 185
Love, Medicine and Miracles, 250
love, need for, 130, 190, 192–194, 221, 222
low-fat diet, 145, 147–148
lymph nodes, 77, 253
lymphatic leukemia, 6, 52, 86–89, 95, 103, 166
lymphedema, 128
lymphoma, 6, 16, 51, 94, 97, 98, 100, 102, 105, 106, 179

lung cancer, xiv, 6, 17, 84, 94, 95, 98, 99, 100, 102, 103, 104, 105, 108, 145, 146

Mack, Robert M., M.D., 197
Magic Mountain, 196
Make Today Count, 176, 144
male sexual issues, 129–130
malignant melanoma, 100
malignant pleural effusions, 98, 104
malignant tumor, 16, 253
malnutrition, 116, 149–150
malnutrition, signs of, 150
mammograms, 38, 75–76, 246
Mann, Thomas, 196
Mantle, Mickey, 4
marijuana, 115, 143
masectomy, 130, 196
Mayo Center, 56
MDR-1 gene, 238
meal preparation tips, 140–142
Meals on Wheels, 140
mechlorethamine (nitrogen mustard et al.), 24, 26, 93, 104, 114, 201
media and cancer, 13, 214–216
Medicaid, 200, 208
medical checkups, returning for, 219–220, 226
medical file, 85, 86, 88, 90, 202
medical history, 37
Medical Information Bureau (MIB),206
medical information, evaluation of, 42, 91
medical misinformation, 211–217
medical oncologists, 24, 67
medical records, 82,85, 86–89, 90, 202
medical specialists, 67–70
medical tests, 38, 48, 60, 171, 200, 219–220
medical treatment team, 63–70
Medicare, 200, 208, 233, 234, 246
Medicare information line, 246
medications for constipation, 125
medications for diarrhea, 124–125
medications for pain relief, 161–164
meditation, 180–181, 213
MEDLARS, 248
MEDLINE, 91, 248

Nixon, Daniel W., M.D., 144
nodule, definition, 253
non-Hodgkin's lymphoma, 98, 99, 100,
    103, 104, 106, 109, 148
noninvasive medical tests, 48
nonlymphocytic leukemia, 102, 108
nonmedical treatment techniques,
    113, 160–161, 179–186
NSAIDs (nonsteroidal, anti-inflamma-
    tory drugs), 162–163
nutrients, depletion of, 136
nutrients, need for additional, 135–136
nutrition, 68, 119, 135–150, 174, 213,
    223, 239
nutritionists, 68, 138–139, 142–143,
    146, 150, 165

obesity, 144
off-label uses of drugs, 202–203
older people, considerations for, 14, 39,
    40, 47, 86–89
Olympic Games, 223
Omodiu, 124
oncogenes, 238
OncoLink, 248
oncologists, 67–68, 253
oncology fellows, 58
oncology nurses, 68, 72, 82–84, 187–188,
    232
Oncovin 26; *also see* vincristine
"one on one" programs, 193
Ontario Cancer Information Service,
    242
open enrollment, 207
organ transplants, 99
orientation sessions, 82
OSHA, 73
osteosarcoma, 52
ostomies, 247
ovarian cancer 6, 26, 49, 85, 96, 98, 99,
    100, 102, 103, 105, 106, 107, 108, 144
overmedication of terminal patients,
    231
"overnutrition," risk factor of, 144–145
overview of contents of book, 7–9
Ovid Technologies, 248
outcomes of treatment, summary of,
    43–44

outpatient issues, 25, 71, 136, 188

package inserts, 202–203
pain, 30, 39, 44, 76–77, 129, 157–164,
    166, 170, 174, 231, 246
    causes of, 158
    clinics for, 165, 254
    how to describe to doctor, 159–160
    incidence of, 157, 174
    ladder of treatment for, 162
    psychological aspects of, 158
    techniques to relieve, 31, 160–161,
    179–186, 229
    undertreatment of, 157
palliation of symptoms 39, 44–45, 161,
    253
palliative surgery, 161–162
pancreatic cancer, 94, 100, 102, 105,
    107, 144
paragoric, 124
Parschan, Richard, Ph.D., 235
partnership with doctor, 2, 64–67, 81
pathologists, 68
patient role in treatment, 63–65, 81–92
"patients active," 167
Pauling, Linus, 146–147
PDQ (Physicians' Data Query), 2, 3, 5,
    41, 61–62, 66, 96, 242
"PEB" regimen, 20
Pedriatic Branch, NCI, NIH, 242
pedriatic cancer, *see* children with
    cancer
pedriatic hospitals, 52
pedriatic oncologists, 51, 68
Pediatric Oncology Group, 58
pedriatic surgeons, 51
Percodan, 162
Peron, Eva, 4
personal advocate, benefits of, 45, 75,
    82
personal imaging programs, 152
personal notebook, 90
personal trainers, 69, 185
pet therapy, 254
Peter's story, 20–22
Petterle, Elmo A., 234
pharmacists, 68, 165
Phase I-III trials, 60

Index

Index